ACUPRESSURE

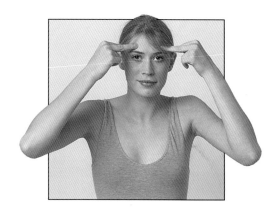

CAROLA BERESFORD-COOKE

PETER ALBRIGHT M.D., SERIES EDITOR

MACMILLAN • USA

ISBN 0-02-860833-X

This book was designed and produced by
Quarto Inc.
The Old Brewery
6 Blundell Street
London N7 9BH
England

Senior editor Sally MacEachern
Editor Alison Leach
Editorial assistant Judith Evans
Indexer Dorothy Frame
Senior art editor Penny Cobb
Designer Alyson Kyles
Picture researcher Susannah Jayes
Illustrators Samantha Elmhurst, Sharon Smith
Photographers Paul Forrester, Colin Bowling
Picture research manager Giulia Hetherington
Editorial director Mark Dartford
Art director Moira Clinch

Typeset by Central Southern Typesetters, Eastbourne
Manufactured in Hong Kong by Regent Publishing Services Ltd
Printed in China by Leefung-Asco Printers Ltd

10 9 8 7 6 5 4 3 2 1

CONTENTS

INTRODUCTION

The chances are that if you have picked up this book out of interest, you will already have some idea about what "acupressure" means. Although the word is a concocted Western term, it does convey the idea of pressure which is in some way connected with acupuncture; and it is a commonly accepted name for pressure-point massage applied according to acupuncture principles. Most people now know of acupuncture as an effective and acceptable "complementary" treatment.

Self-acupressure is a safe and easy way to help many everyday complaints.

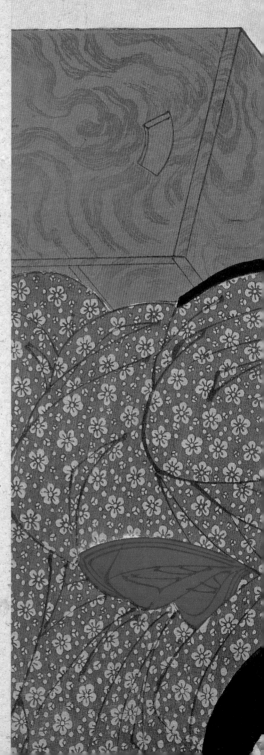

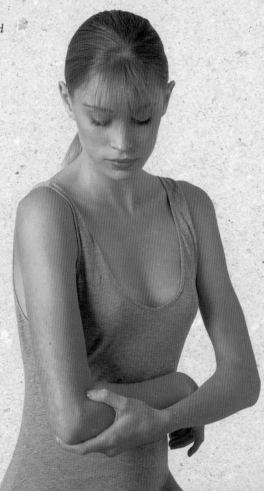

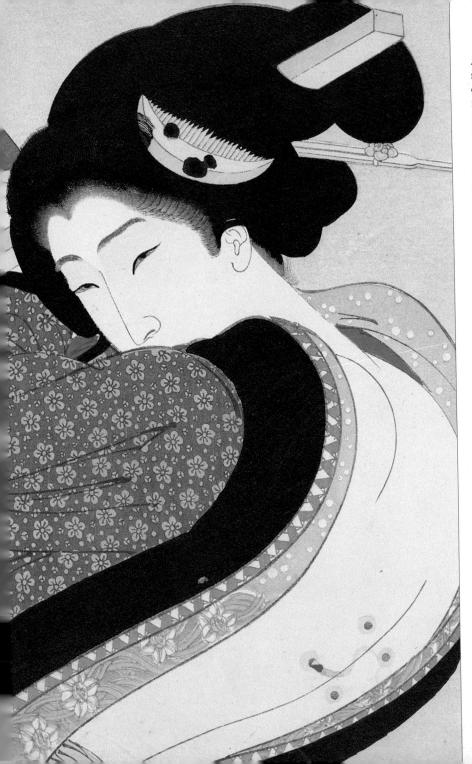

Acupressure, as you will find if you read further and decide to try it, is as effective and more pleasurable to receive, and of course it makes much more sense as a form of self-treatment. But how does it work? The theory which lies behind both acupuncture and acupressure remains a mystery to the Western scientific mind. Imagine a system of medicine which links the condition of the human body to everything that surrounds it – to the weather and seasons, to the plant and mineral worlds, to colors and sounds, to emotional influences. Although it sounds unscientific, the concept of such a medical system strikes a chord in many people. After all, some diseases are stress-related, and thus linked to the emotions; many people have experienced a physical condition that is linked to the season or weather. Oriental medicine relates human beings to their environment and to the complex mixture of heredity, behavior habits, and lifestyle which makes each person unique. It does not see humans as made up of separate systems and replaceable parts.

WHY DOES ACUPRESSURE WORK?

Until recently, Western scientists have been suggesting that acupuncture's effectiveness as a treatment for pain may be related to the blocking of pain-gates in the spinal cord and the simultaneous release of endorphins. However, as the technique continues to prove effective for conditions other than pain, such as nausea, this explanation may no longer apply. A newer, exciting theory suggests that acupuncture's effectiveness may be related to the transfer of information between body parts and systems via the fascia, or connective tissue.

The fascia is a semitransparent, almost luminous, tough covering which surrounds every muscle, joint, blood-vessel, bone, and organ in the body. The continuity of this tissue extends to the lining of the spinal cord and of the brain, and a layer of superficial fascia runs under the surface of the skin. If you have seen a cut of uncooked meat, you will have seen the fascia in its natural state, a crystalline white membrane. A large number of acupuncture meridians – the channels connecting the points – lie along fascial planes, areas where two layers of fascia rub together.

As the fibers of the fascia are similar to crystals in structure, and since pressure on crystals creates a kind of electricity known as piezo-electricity, the theory is that pressure along the acupuncture meridians and on the acupuncture points generates a type of electric current, which causes signals to run through the network of fascia to tissues a long distance from the site of the pressure. This ties in with the fact (already established through research) that acupressure points have a lower electrical resistance than the surrounding tissues.

There is a long way to go in research, and there is little incentive for funding such research, since there is minimal or no profit to be expected as a result. Acupressure practitioners, however, know that it is only a matter of time before Western scientific research catches up with the principles that were first established in China about 6,000 years ago.

It was in tombs dating from that time that the first acupuncture needles (stone ones!) were found. Since stone needles cannot penetrate far into body tissues, it can be assumed that the needles were used as an aid to deeper pressure in acupressure techniques. In fact, it makes sense to conclude that acupressure came before acupuncture – pressing and rubbing a point that relieves pain is something that we all do instinctively.

A Complete Medical System

It is often assumed that acupuncture and acupressure constitute the whole of Oriental medicine, but actually such practices are only part of a complete medical system which originated in China long ago. The four main branches of Chinese medicine are herbalism, acupuncture, moxibustion (deep heat applied to points on the body by means of burning powdered mugwort), and massage, which would once have included bone-setting and manipulation as well as massage techniques and acupressure. Other off-shoots are dietary therapy, special forms of exercise such as Qi Gong, and breathing techniques.

Attention to principles of health governs the Oriental lifestyle to a great extent; there is respect for the natural rhythms of the body and an awareness of environmental influences. The emphasis is on prevention of disease through harmonizing the body with the environment, both physically and emotionally, externally and internally.

The medical system which originated in China spread throughout the Far East, and each country has modified the system according to its

You can use acupressure to help family and friends, as it has been used in Far Eastern cultures since time immemorial.

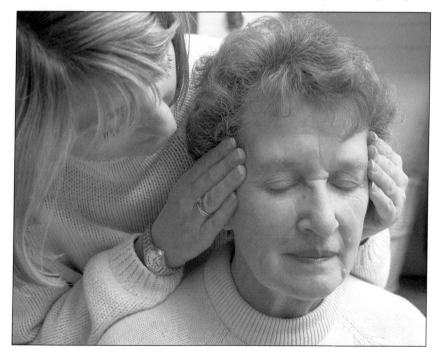

unique environment and culture. There are forms of pressure-point massage in Japan, Korea, Tibet, southern India, Indonesia, Thailand, and the Philippines. In most of these countries, acupressure is practiced between family members and friends as a form of folk medicine for everyday ailments, but there are professional practitioners, too. It is often practiced by blind people, whose developed sense of touch assists them in locating points.

Principle of Qi

The principle behind the use of points and meridians is that of Qi (pronounced "Chi"), which can be loosely translated as "energy," a word which only gives half the picture. The Chinese character for Qi includes the symbol for "steam" and the symbol for "rice," indicating that Qi is both insubstantial and substantial; it is activity within the body tissues and their ability to adapt to changing circumstances. On another level, it could be said that Qi also represents the interface where mind and body meet. A person's Qi is influenced in specific ways by the emotions as well as by diet, occupation, weather, and ancestry.

Although Qi functions throughout the body, there are specific pathways – the meridians or channels – within which Qi flows from place to place. They are like supply lines of Qi. Along them are the points, which influence the quality of Qi and of the other body substances associated with it, such as the blood, and which increase or reduce the flow of Qi to the various body parts. Some points can also expel dangerous forms of Qi which attack the body from outside – these external forms of Qi are associated with climatic factors such as

cold, wind, heat, or damp, and often correspond to bacterial or viral illnesses in Western terms. In China, various massage techniques such as cupping are used, as well as points, in order to grasp and remove the "external pathogenic Qi."

In the East, acupressure is often given routinely as a preventive measure against disease. In Japan, for instance, the local version of acupressure, Shiatsu (meaning "finger-pressure"), is often offered by large firms to their employees in order to reduce stress and minimize absenteeism. It can be used in this way in the West, too, and more and more people have regular acupressure or Shiatsu treatments because of the sense of well-being and relaxation which results from a balanced flow of Qi. For information on how to find a practitioner, turn to pages 60-1.

Use in Everyday Ailments

In the Far East, Grandmother's rheumatism, Dad's hangover, Mom's headache, and the baby's cold will all be treated with a few acupressure points as well as with the traditional herbal and dietary remedies that survive in folklore. As state systems of health-care become more overloaded and private medicine more expensive, self-help is becoming as popular in the West as it has always been in the East. This is where this book can help you.

You will probably want to use the acupressure points on yourself at first, to find out where they are, and if they work for you. Or you may also feel like using the points and techniques to help a friend, and simple instructions are included on how to do this. The points can be combined with orthodox medication, and with other systems of

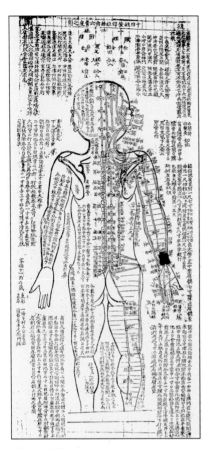

The meridians are the pathways through which Qi flows in the body, and the points are "command stations" where the Qi can be influenced.

complementary medicine such as aromatherapy, homeopathy, and herbal remedies. Where relevant, simple health-care advice is included with the points in the Specific Applications section (pages 48-59).

Acupressure can be a way of caring for yourself in a very practical and effective way, provided the basic principles (pages 8-11) are followed. I hope you enjoy using this book.

BASIC PRINCIPLES

Before you begin discovering how to improve your health and energy with acupressure, remind yourself of a few commonsense guidelines. Always remember that acupressure is complementary to, not a substitute for, medical care. Do not use acupressure to treat your symptoms, or anyone else's, unless they have been diagnosed by a doctor. What may seem an everyday ailment could be a symptom of a more serious condition requiring professional treatment. It is possible to use acupressure at the same time as orthodox medication, but you should never stop taking any prescribed medication without the approval of your doctor.

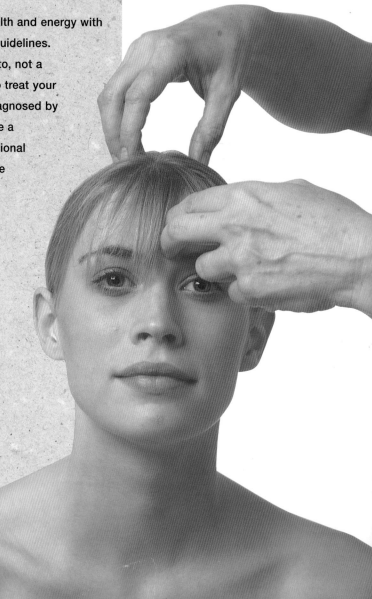

Acupressure can and should be a pleasurable experience for both giver and receiver when it is approached in a relaxed frame of mind.

FINDING THE POINTS

Clear instructions on how to find the points are given in the text, so try to follow them as precisely as possible. The points are often placed in hollows or next to bony protuberances which are easy to find. Or, you can measure the distance between the point and the nearest bony landmark using the width of your thumb or fingers as a measurement. When you are sure you are within millimeters of the point, you can begin exploring for the precise location and angle. Most points, when pressed, give a characteristic sensation, a dull ache which spreads beyond the point itself. This ache often feels in some way pleasurable. However, even if it is not, the pain should never be sharp or excessive.

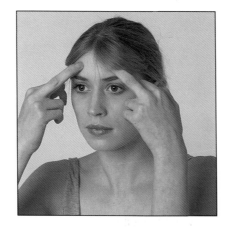

Observe your own sensations as a guideline of where best to apply pressure.

If you do not feel much of a sensation, avoid poking around until the area is sore; instead, try changing the angle of your pressure. Classically, the pressure should be directed toward the area of your problem, but you may find that some other direction of pressure finds the point. Use your sensations as a guide. The same principles apply to working with a partner, but you will then need a good deal of verbal feedback. Remember, too, that everyone has very different ways of experiencing and describing sensation, and that the different points can produce different sensations in the same person.

PRESSING THE POINTS

How to press is very much up to you, especially when working on your own body. You will find out what works best for you as you go along.

1 As a basic guide, after you've located the point and the angle of pressure, relax and press in gradually, holding and concentrating on the point for 5–10 seconds.

2 Release the point, and then immediately press in again for the same time. This prevents you from losing concentration, and also prevents the point from becoming numb.

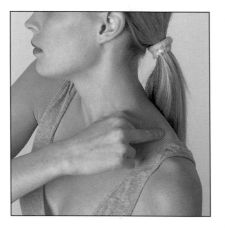

3 Repeat the pressure until you have pressed and released five times. Then do the same point on the other side of the body (all points except those on the midline are bilateral).

CAUTIONS

• Do not use acupressure on the sites of unhealed fractures or on areas where the skin is broken. If using a point which lies on a scar, especially on the chest or abdomen, use only gentle pressure.
• Do not press directly on varicose veins on the legs.
• Do not use acupressure if you have a fever.
• Do not use it on areas which are inflamed (hot, red, swollen, painful).
• Do not use very hard pressure on anyone (including yourself) with high blood pressure or osteoporosis.
• Do not press breast or other glandular tissue, such as lymph glands.
• Finally, do observe the contra-indications for certain points in pregnancy.

RELAXATION

When you are finding and treating a point, you will get much better results if you remain relaxed. Sensory information flows better through relaxed muscles and tissues, so relax the area you are treating, and the hand you are pressing with, and make yourself comfortable with supporting pillows. If you follow the instructions (right) for breathing and visualization, you will find that you need relatively little physical pressure to achieve quite a strong sensation.

• Use the tip of your thumb or finger and try to find a comfortable posture which does not place your hand or arm in a sharp angle.

• Never use physical force to obtain a sensation. Your maximum pressure should be about 15 pounds – try it on your bathroom scales. Any greater pressure will bruise the tissues, strain your thumb, and be quite unnecessary. Lighter pressure usually works fine.

This point can help clear blocked sinuses even better if you visualize a light beam traveling up from the point to your face and clearing the area.

BREATHING, FOCUS, AND VISUALIZATION

There is a saying, as old as Chinese medicine, that "the Mind rules the Qi," and you can put this principle to work in making your use of points more effective.

As you press a point, try to "think beyond" the surface of the skin. Imagine that there is a tiny laser beam at the end of your thumb or finger which is traveling right through the body tissues and out the other side. Stay relaxed, though! This works whether it is your own body or someone else's that you are pressing. It is a variation on a technique used to great effect in the martial arts, except that in acupressure it is used for

healing purposes. As you gain in experience and confidence, you can work with sending the "laser beam" from the point you are pressing to the area you want to help.

When you are using a point for a specific complaint – for example, if you are using a point on your wrist to help nausea, use your breathing as well. Having found and contacted the point, slow your breathing down if it is rapid and, as you breathe in, imagine a pathway between the sensation in the point on your wrist and the area in your stomach where you feel the nausea, as if you were breathing in from your wrist to your stomach. As you breathe out, imagine the nauseous sensation leaving you along with the spent breath.

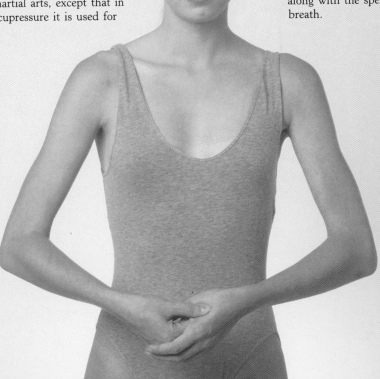

MASSAGE ROUTINES

Although the acupressure points for dealing with a physical problem are often a long distance from the area of the problem, one of the Chinese acupressure techniques is to disperse accumulated or "stagnant" Qi in the area itself with a pressure massage routine. For example, if you have blocked sinuses, you can use a point on your hand to help disperse them, but the messages sent through this point will get through much more easily if you help to decongest the tissues and clear the drainage passages with a massage routine for your face as well. Routines for four main areas are given in detail on pages 26-36, but you can just as well improvise your own, once you are familiar with the technique. Anything that "feels right" to you (and to your partner, if you are working with one) will probably do good, so do follow your intuition, it will help you to follow the Qi!

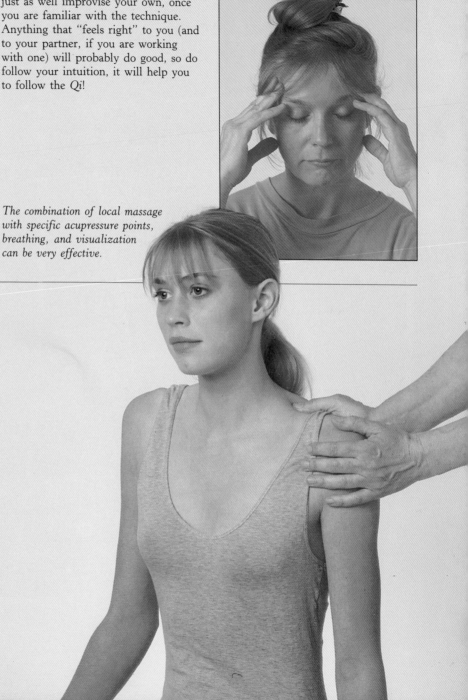

The combination of local massage with specific acupressure points, breathing, and visualization can be very effective.

WORKING WITH A PARTNER

All the principles which apply to using the points on yourself will also help you to work on a friend. The principles are the same, although finding the points needs quite a lot of feedback from your partner; otherwise, relax, breathe, and visualize (and get your friend to do so, too!) exactly as described above. There are detailed instructions on how to work with a partner on pages 38-47.

The healing power of acupressure can be even more effective for a friend.

THE POINTS

The network of acupressure meridians is a subtle and complex system extending throughout the body. In Western physiological terms, it has links with the nervous system as well as with the connective tissues and fascia. Many of the points along the meridians, although not all of them, correspond with the "trigger" points used in physiotherapy to release tight muscles. The points are not always in exactly the same position on everyone, since meridians can become distorted by injury or long-term postural habits; so do persevere when trying to find them, and explore the area about an inch around where the point should be if you don't find it the first time.

There are twelve main meridians throughout the body, each influencing the function of a major organ or body system.

POINTS ON THE FOOT AND LEG

The points on the foot and leg can be very powerful in their effect on the reproductive, digestive, and urinary systems. They can be tricky to reach, though. Try sitting in a chair with one leg balanced across your other knee for the points on the inner surface of the leg. For the points on the outer surface, sit in a chair with your foot flat on the floor and bend down to reach the points.

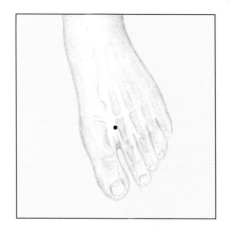

LIVER 3

On the top of the foot, in the "V" between the bones leading to the big toe and the second toe (the first and second metatarsals). Try pressing the

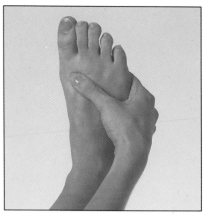

sole at the same time, using your thumb and index finger in a pinching movement.

Commonly used for problems anywhere in the body linked with tension, emotional stress, or frustration.

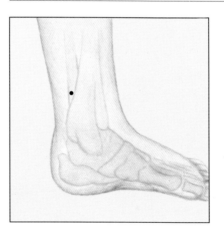

SPLEEN 6

On the inside of the leg, four fingers' width above the tip of the ankle bone, in the groove behind the shin bone.

One of the most important points in the body. Relaxes and soothes, helps

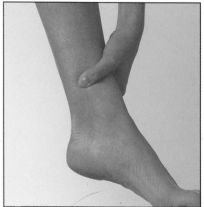

the body absorb nourishment, stimulates and tones the digestive system, and helps problems in the lower part of the body. Has a special affinity with the female reproductive system, toning the uterus. *Contra-indicated in pregnancy.*

SPLEEN 9

In the groove behind the shin bone, on the inner surface of the leg just below the bulge at the top of the bone, about three fingers' width below the level of the knee crease.

Often very tender, especially in women. Frequently used to expel fluid retention in the lower part of the body.

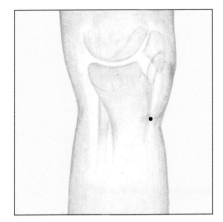 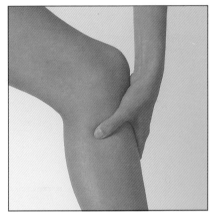

STOMACH 36

On the front of the leg, four fingers' width below the bottom edge of the kneecap (you need to feel carefully for this) and one finger's width to the outside of the shin bone.

Tonifies the whole body via the digestive system, increasing energy and reducing fatigue. Also relieves digestive problems and increases resistance to disease.

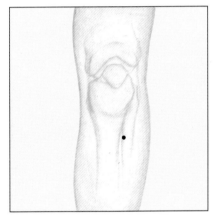 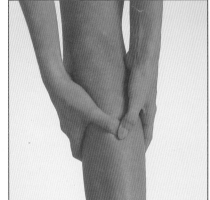

STOMACH 44

On the web of flesh between the second and third toes, at the base of the second toe where it joins the body of the foot. Press toward the base of the second toe.

Has a cooling effect, not only on a hot, irritated digestive system, but also on the stomach meridian, which goes to the head and jaw.

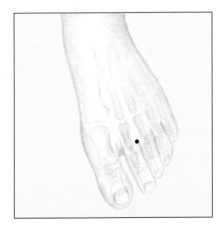 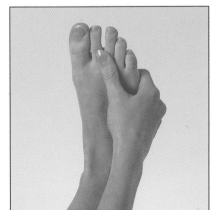

KIDNEY 3

Level with the tip of the inner ankle bone and halfway between it and the Achilles tendon.

Restores balance between the ability to act and the ability to relax – energizes or soothes, whichever is more appropriate. Strengthens and tonifies the lower back, kidneys, and reproductive system.

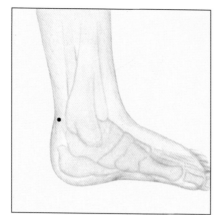

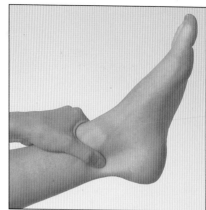

KIDNEY 6

Place the widest part of your thumb under the tip of your inner ankle bone. Having measured the width of your thumb directly down from the tip of the bone, feel for a shallow hollow between two tendons which gives a sensation when pressed. Very important for accessing the body's capacity to accept and maintain the yin properties of relaxation, calm, coolness, and moisture. Also helps build and maintain reserves of essential nutrients.

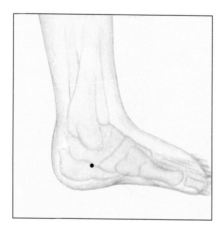

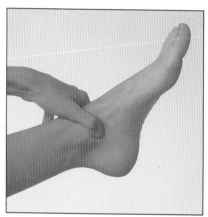

BLADDER 60

Level with the tip of the outer ankle bone and halfway between it and the Achilles tendon.

A point with a strong influence on the area of the spine, from the lower back to the nape of the neck and back of the head. Also benefits the bladder and uterus.

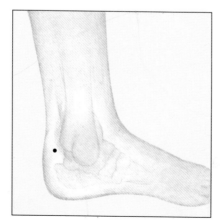

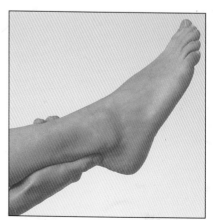

POINTS ON THE TORSO

Points on the torso influence the main organs of the body directly and can be very useful for abdominal and chest complaints, though sometimes they can be quite painful in acute conditions. Do be guided by common sense when you use them. If they cause "grateful pain" and bring relief, they are appropriate to use; if they cause pain and seem not to relieve the condition, do not use them until the acute stage of the problem has subsided.

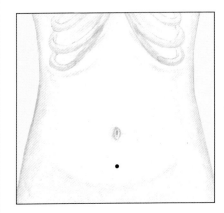

CONCEPTION VESSEL (CV) 6

On the midline of the abdomen, about two fingers' width below the center of the navel. If there is fatty tissue here, try jiggling your finger or thumb very slightly as you begin to press, in order to embed it as much as possible in the muscular layer of the abdomen.

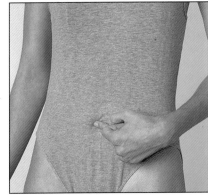

Another generally tonifying point for the whole body. The area below the navel has a special significance in Oriental medicine as the center of the body's stored resources or energy. Tai Chi or martial arts practitioners know this area as the Dan Tian or the Hara.

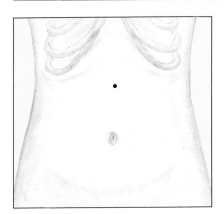

CONCEPTION VESSEL (CV) 12

Feel up both sides of your rib cage until you find where they meet. The point is halfway between the meeting of your ribs and your navel. Make sure

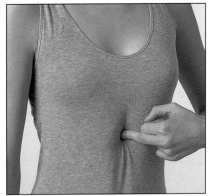

you measure the distance accurately. Press straight in; you may need to jiggle slightly first, as for CV 6. Tonifies and regulates the digestive system.

CONCEPTION VESSEL (CV) 17

On the breastbone, halfway between the nipples (this applies on a man; in a woman, you must estimate where the nipples would be if the breasts were pressed flat to the chest like a man's).

Energizes and clears the whole chest area, helps breathing and benefits the diaphragm.

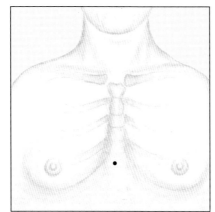
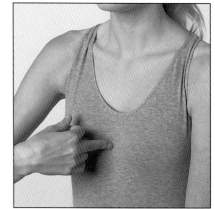

CONCEPTION VESSEL (CV) 22

At the top of the breastbone, in the bony notch halfway between the collar-bones, where the breastbone meets the throat. Do not press inward; you could damage the windpipe. Press vertically down into the bony notch.

Used to clear and soothe the throat and chest.

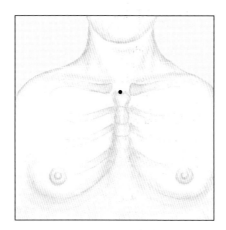
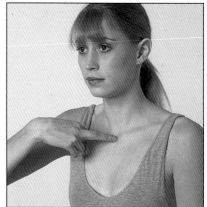

STOMACH 25

On the abdomen, three fingers' width on each side of the navel. Press straight in.

Regulates the Qi of the intestines and is helpful in many intestinal problems, especially diarrhea.

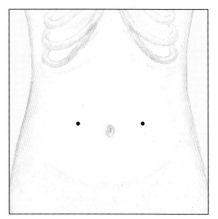
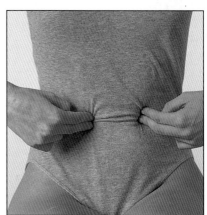

LIVER 13

Place your hands on your hips in a natural way, with your fingers curving around the front of your waist. Your index finger will be approximately level with the bottom of your rib cage; if you press into the flesh just above your waistline, you will find the free end of your eleventh rib curving around to the front of your body. The point is just underneath it. Press straight in.

Has a powerful effect on digestive troubles, particularly those which are stress-related.

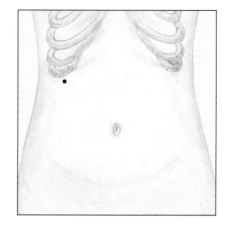

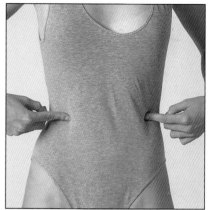

LUNG 1

Feel along the bottom edge of your collarbone, outward from the midline of your body. A natural valley between the chest wall and the shoulder joint reaches its deepest point in a small hollow under the collarbone. The point is about an inch directly below this hollow and is very often tender under pressure.

The main action of this point is to clear a stuffy or congested chest and relieve coughs.

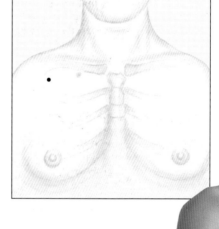

This is the point which is treated indirectly in the partner routine on page 45 by leaning on the shoulders. It is good for "opening" stooped shoulders caused by poor breathing.

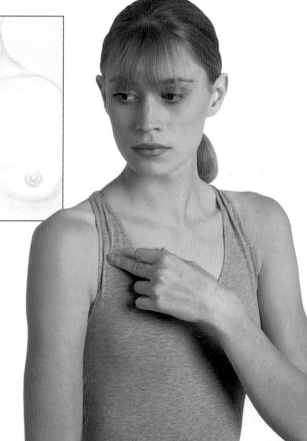

POINTS ON THE ARM AND HAND

Points on the arm and hand influence the chest and throat, and are thus mainly used for circulatory and respiratory conditions. Try to sit upright but relaxed, and avoid tensing up your shoulders and arms as you press. Visualization and breathing are particularly helpful with these points.

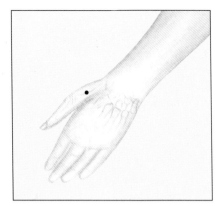

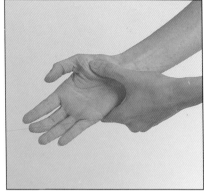

LUNG 10

Find the bone that connects your wrist and your thumb (the first metacarpal) and measure halfway along the bone from joint to joint. Using this halfway mark as a guideline, move around to the fleshy part of the thumb pad, where the point is located.

Has a cooling action on the chest and throat, and is particularly good for sore, inflamed throats.

LUNG 9

On the wrist crease, at the base of the thumb, where a pulse can be felt. Don't press directly on the artery! Move very slightly to one side of it, bend your wrist slightly to find the gap between the bones and angle your pressure into that gap and down toward your thumb.

Tonifies the lungs and is good to use regularly if you suffer from lots of colds or have a chronic cough or sore throat. Also good for the circulation.

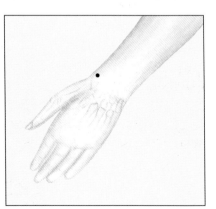

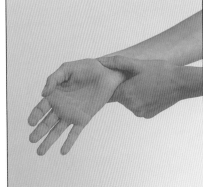

LUNG 7

On the inner surface of the forearm, about two fingers' width along from Lung 9.

A very important point for use at the very beginning of a cold or flu, especially in conjunction with Large Intestine 4 (opposite). It repels infection.

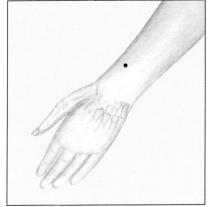
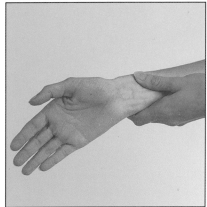

LUNG 5

In the elbow crease, in line with Lung 9 and the thumb. Bend your elbow so that you can angle your pressure deep into the hollow.

The point for phlegm in the lungs. If you have a rattly or "wet" cough, or cough up lots of phlegm, this is the point to use.

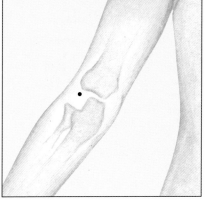

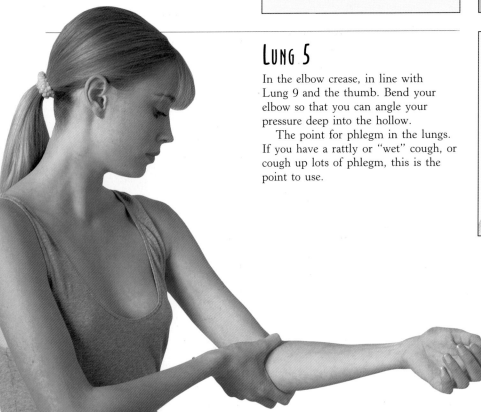

Breathing "into" this point while pressing it can really help a phlegmy cough.

LARGE INTESTINE 4

On the back of the hand, on the web of flesh between thumb and first finger, in the "V" between the bones. Considered to have a strong expelling action, hence its contraindication in pregnancy.

Used chiefly in expelling infections, particularly those affecting the eyes, nose, mouth, and face. The point of choice at the beginning of a cold or flu. Often used in conjunction with Liver 3 (page 13) to reduce pain and calm anxiety. *Contraindicated in pregnancy.*

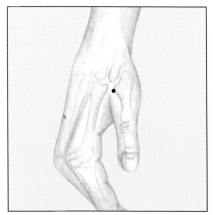 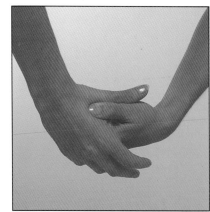

LARGE INTESTINE 10

If you bend your arm across your chest, you can look down at this point. It is on a line running between the elbow crease and the index finger, on the bulge of the arm muscle, three fingers' width below the elbow crease.

Much used throughout the Far East for increasing stamina and well-being. Also used for muscular problems of the arm and hand.

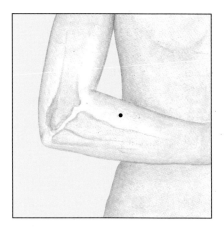 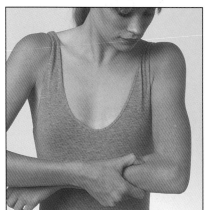

LARGE INTESTINE 11

Bend your arm across your chest. The point is at the end of the elbow crease. Angle your pressure down into the joint.

A cooling point. Obviously used for fevers and other conditions where there is evident heat, but can also be used for problems such as high blood pressure, or red and itchy skin conditions. Can also help with tennis elbow.

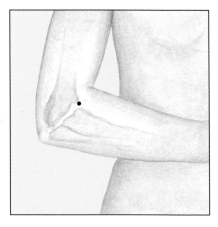 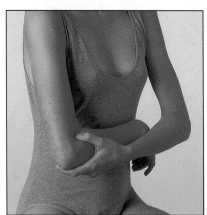

HEART 7

On the wrist crease, directly below the little finger, there is a bony lump (the pisiform bone) to which a tendon is attached. The point lies under the tendon and, in some people, slightly under the bone, so angle your pressure backward and under it.

Not so much a point for heart problems (although it is a safe and gentle one to use if you do have a heart condition) as a calming and soothing point for anxiety and stress.

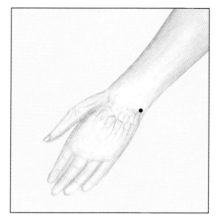

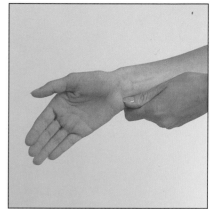

ACUPRESSURE "WRISTBAND"

These wristbands are now widely available for treating travel sickness and can sometimes be helpful for morning sickness in pregnancy.

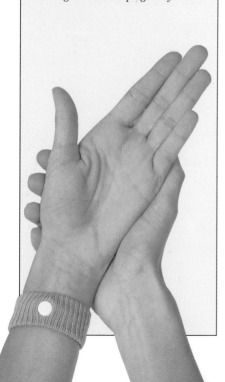

PERICARDIUM 6

Measure three fingers' width up the inner surface of the arm from the middle of the wrist crease. The point lies between two tendons which can be felt if the hand is clenched.

This is the famous point for travel sickness for which special "acupressure wristbands" are sold. In addition to its scientifically proven usefulness for nausea of all kinds, it is very helpful for pain in the chest and is a calming point for anxiety and insomnia.

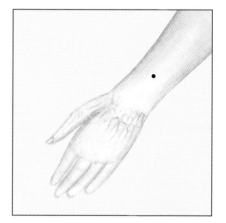

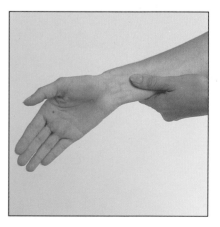

Points on the Face, Neck, and Shoulders

Points on the neck, face, and shoulders can feel wonderful. Their long-term effectiveness is limited, however, unless you use them in combination with other points or recommendations; they are more in the nature of first-aid points for immediate relief of symptoms (see page 51).

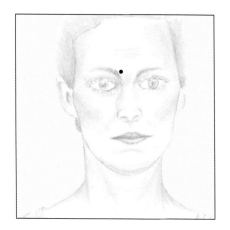

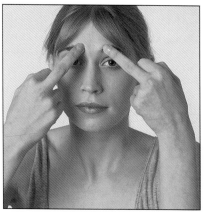

Bladder 2

On the thickest part of the eyebrow, at the inner end.

The Chinese name of this point is "Collect Bamboo." Used for hay fever, which must have made it useful on bamboo-gathering expeditions in ancient China!

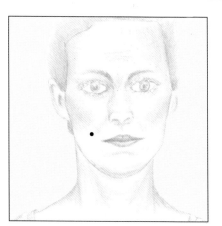

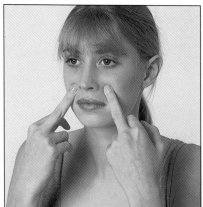

Stomach 3

On the laughter line, in line with the pupil of the eye when the eye is looking straight ahead. Press up under the cheekbone.

Used for eye and nose problems, facial tics, and sinusitis. In my experience, it is also a calming and soothing point.

LARGE INTESTINE 20

At the point where the "laughter lines" meet the nose, level with the midpoint of the nostril. Press straight in toward the face.

Use for any kind of nose problems. Traditionally, you press away from the nostril to clear a blocked nose, and toward it to stop a runny nose.

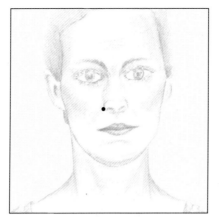

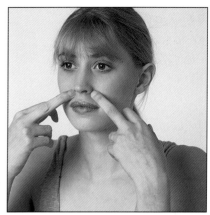

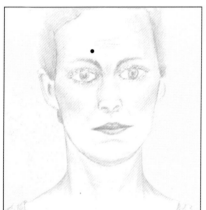

This point is very helpful when used in combination with Gall Bladder 20.

GALL BLADDER 14

Measure halfway along your eyebrow. The point is one-third of the distance up from the midpoint of your eyebrow to your hairline. A helpful point for tension headaches related to eyestrain.

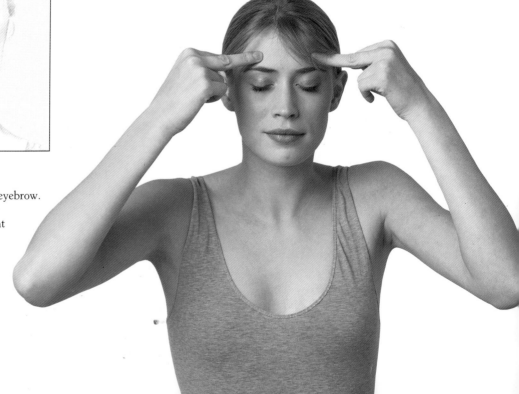

Gall-bladder 20

At the back of the neck, under the base of the skull, halfway between the ear and the midline, in a hollow in the neck muscles. Press slightly upward and toward the opposite eye.

Has many uses, such as relieving colds, headaches, and eye problems. Also helpful for stress-related tension in the shoulders and neck.

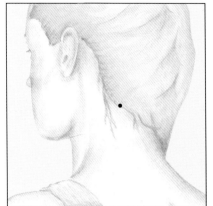 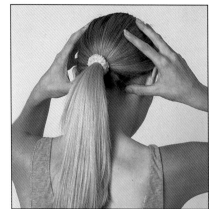

Gall-bladder 21

With your fingertips, press from the base of your neck along the ridge of muscle on the very top of your shoulder. About halfway between your neck and the bones of the shoulder joint, this point is very tender on most people. On someone else, measure half the distance between the big vertebra at the back of the neck and the tip of the shoulder – remember that the point is right on top of the muscle. *Contra-indicated in pregnancy.*

Has a strong downward movement, which makes it a good one to use at the moment when a baby is on its way out of the womb. (But not before that in pregnancy!) Much used to send *Qi* downward away from the shoulders, thus relieving neck and shoulder tension and calming an overburdened mind.

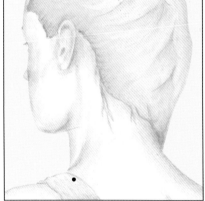

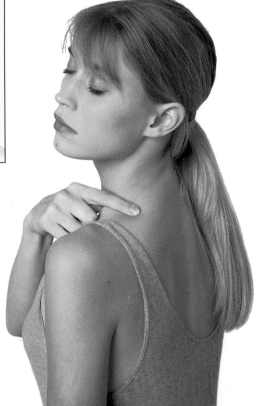

This point needs strong vertical pressure to be effective, especially if your shoulders are very tense. You may find it more useful to use several fingers together when pressing.

PRESSURE MASSAGE ROUTINES

All these routines are variants on forms taken from the most ancient Eastern therapy of all, *Dao Yin*. This combination of self-acupressure, massage, and stretching traveled centuries ago from China to Japan, where its name became *Do-In* and where it is still much practiced. Do make yourself comfortable before performing the routines, so that you are as relaxed as possible.

Self-massage is a way of being kind to yourself. Approached in this frame of mind, a self-massage routine can help restore inner harmony and balance.

RELAXATION TECHNIQUES

Try to make the pressure massage routines part of a special time for your own needs. A soothing bath beforehand and some favorite music playing will help you to unwind so that the massage is more effective; try to allow yourself some relaxation time afterward, too.

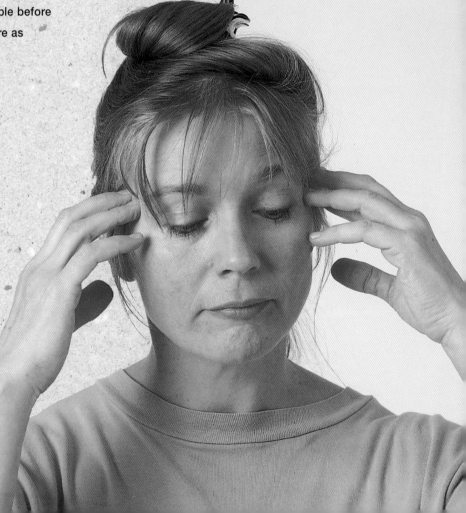

FACE ROUTINE

The sequences in this routine will ease tension, help drain sinuses and nasal passages, help to keep your teeth and gums healthy, and help to keep you looking good. The fingertips of a relaxed hand are your best pressure tool for this routine, and it is best done in a sitting position. Wherever possible, drop your face onto your hands and let the weight of your head do the work. Don't move or circle with the pressure; and try to imagine that you are penetrating through the tissues themselves, rather than just pressing on the surface.

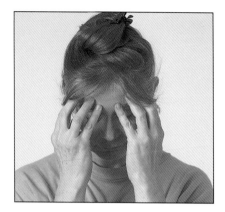

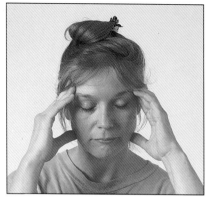

FOREHEAD PRESSURE

Separate your fingers slightly, and let them form a natural curve. Place the tips of your fingers on your forehead, near the hairline, and let your head fall forward slightly so that your fingertips press gently into your forehead. Cover your whole forehead with pressures, working from the center out and the top down.

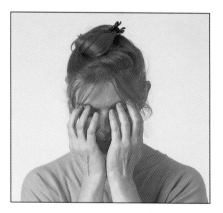

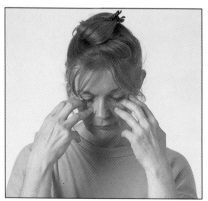

AROUND THE EYE SOCKET

Bring your fingers a little closer together and place them along the ridge of bone you can feel just above your eyelid crease. Very gently, using the weight of your head, press your fingertips into the edge of this bone, working from the inner part near the nose to the outer corner of the eye. When you have finished the upper eye socket, place your fingers on the ridge of bone just below the eye. *Very gently,* press down onto this ridge, working outward from the nose in the same way.

CHEEK PRESSURES

Separate your fingers a little more widely and, working from the nose out, apply pressures to the cheeks (both at once) in the same way as the forehead. When you come to the lower part of the cheeks, follow the ridge of the cheekbone, and press up under the bone all the way around.

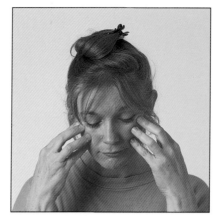
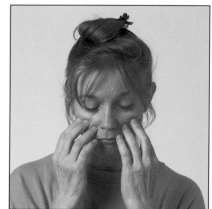

JAW PRESSURES

With your fingertips a little closer together, apply pressures around the top of your mouth, working from the center out. This is one time when it is all right to circle your fingers around a little, so that you massage your upper gums through the flesh. Make sure you can feel the pressure in your gums.

Then, supporting your chin with your thumbs, begin applying fingertip pressures from the center out along your lower jaw in the same way, massaging in tiny circles as long as you can feel your gums. Move your thumbs along, supporting your jawbone gently as you go, and apply firmer fingertip pressure without circling as you leave the mouth area and approach the big jaw muscles. As you reach the corner of the jaw, carry your pressures (slightly more gently) up in front of your ears and finish with a long, gentle pressure on your temples.

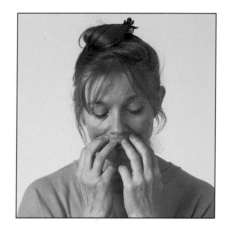
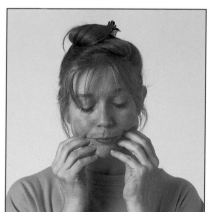
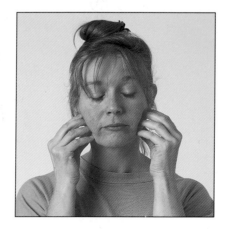
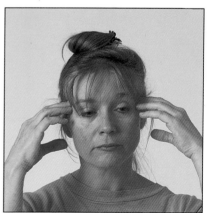

SCALP PRESSURES

Place your fingertips on your scalp at the hairline of your forehead. Press gently, curving your fingers so that you are almost hooking into the scalp, and remember to press *beyond* the surface. Move your hands back so that you are pressing in lines along the top of your head. Then place your fingertips on your hairline at the temples, and press back along the sides of your head in the same manner. Finally, place your fingertips at the back hairline behind your ears and work toward the crown of your head so that you cover the back part of your scalp.

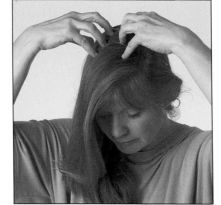

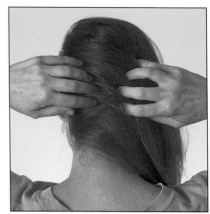

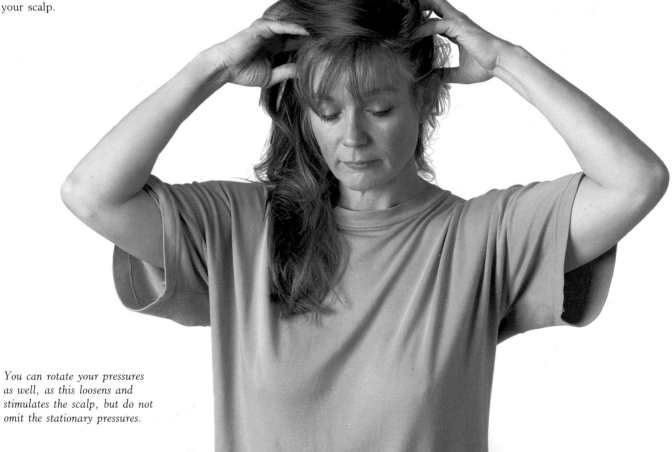

You can rotate your pressures as well, as this loosens and stimulates the scalp, but do not omit the stationary pressures.

NECK AND SHOULDERS ROUTINE

This is a great de-stressing routine, particularly if combined with your favorite parts from the Face Routine. You can be firmer with these movements. The traditional form includes some thumping with the fists, but here is a version you will find more user-friendly. A sitting position in a backless or low-backed chair is best for this routine.

It is important to relax your shoulders while pressing these points, focusing your attention on your breathing helps.

PRESSURE AROUND THE BASE OF THE SKULL

Locate the bony lumps behind your ears, and find the groove underneath them. With your elbows up high and your fingers spread out on the side of your head for support, press your thumbs straight into this groove, moving with repeated pressures under the base of your skull toward the center of the back of your neck. The extreme back of your neck will be hard to reach with your thumbs, so stop when the movement begins to feel awkward.

Keep your head upright or tilted very slightly forward as you press.

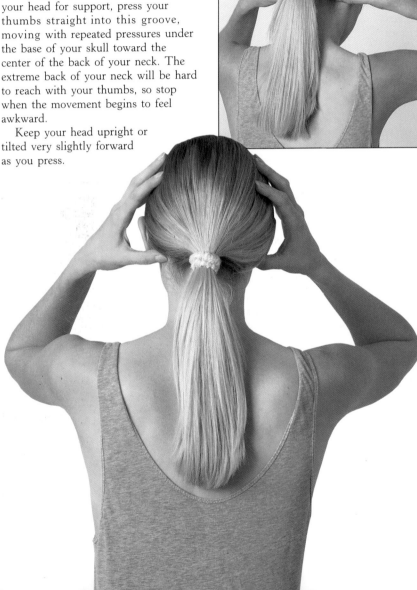

GRASPING THE BACK OF THE NECK

Cup your stronger hand (i.e., right if you are right-handed) horizontally over the upper part of the back of the neck, the part that was awkward to reach with your thumbs. Cup your other hand directly over it. You will find that you are grasping the central muscles of the back of the neck.

Using both hands together for stronger pressure, squeeze the muscle with grasping movements all the way down to the base of your neck.

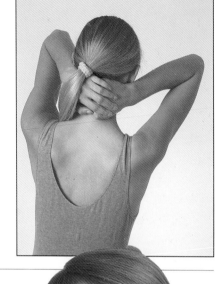

CIRCLES DOWN THE SIDES OF THE NECK

This movement is more effective if you *don't* turn your head to the side. Place the fingers of one hand flat on your neck, under the ear on the *opposite* side. Slowly and deeply circle your fingers around, moving the tissues without sliding your fingers over the skin surface.

Move the circles slowly down the side of the neck. Hook your fingertips in slightly if it feels good. Repeat with the other hand on the other side.

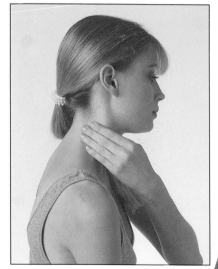

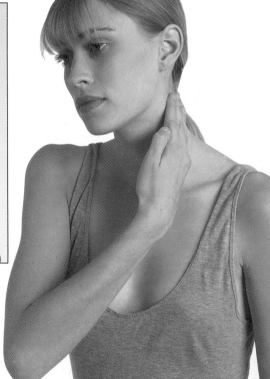

Grasping Shoulders and Upper Arms

Place one hand on the top of the opposite shoulder, close to your neck. Using the heel of your hand and your fingertips (which are reaching onto the back of your shoulder), grasp and squeeze the muscles. Repeat the squeezing movement while moving farther out toward the tip of your shoulder. Go easy over the bony shoulder joint, but increase your pressure again as you move out on to the muscles of the arm. Grasp firmly to halfway down the upper arm. Repeat on the other side with the other hand.

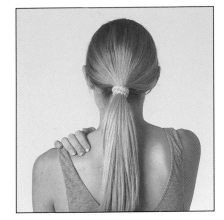
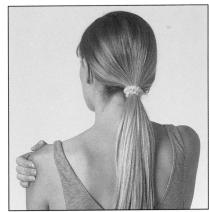

Pressure on Upper Back

Place one hand over your opposite shoulder with your fingertips on your upper back, next to the big vertebra at the base of your neck. Press in a line down the side of the spine as far as you can comfortably reach, then return to the top of your back and move your fingers an inch or so outward, away from the spine, and repeat.

Keep on covering your upper back with lines of pressure until you find yourself working the line next to the shoulder blade. Then repeat the whole sequence with the other hand on the opposite side.

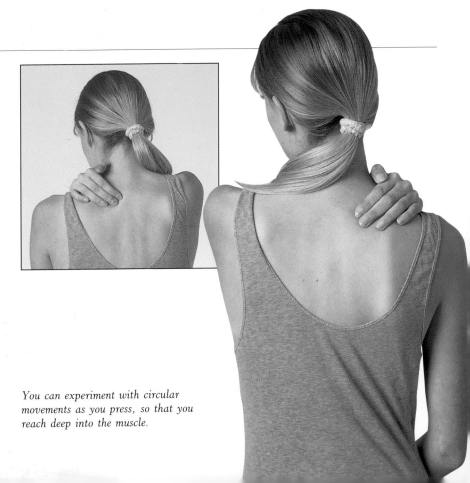

You can experiment with circular movements as you press, so that you reach deep into the muscle.

FINGERTIPS ON CHEST

It may seem strange to include this movement in a sequence for the neck and shoulders, but tension in the upper back and shoulders is so often connected with poor posture that this straightening and opening sequence for the chest is nearly always helpful.

Place your fingertips along the midline of your upper chest, in the center of the breastbone, then move them toward the opposite shoulder until you can feel the beginnings of the ribs. Separating your fingers so that each finger occupies a space between the ribs, press in vertically where the ribs meet the breastbone, and continue pressing out across the chest, keeping your fingers more or less in line, until you reach the arm.

Remember to penetrate beyond the body surface, as if you were reaching into your chest cavity, and observe your sensations. If any area or point feels significant, pay special attention to it. Finish the sequence by pressing with your fingertips or thumb out along the bottom edge of your collarbone, from the midline to the shoulder joint. Repeat the whole sequence on the other side of the chest with the other hand.

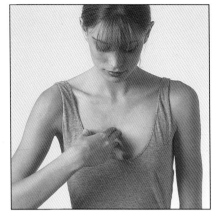
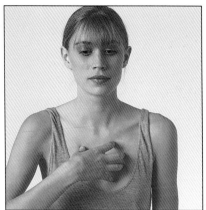
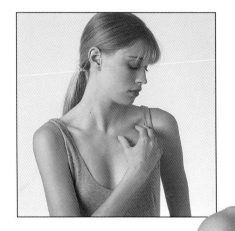

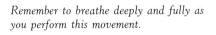

Remember to breathe deeply and fully as you perform this movement.

ABDOMINAL ROUTINE

Abdominal massage, called *Ampuku* in Japan, is one of the most effective techniques of the acupressure or Shiatsu practitioner. Even if you don't take to the idea of massaging your stomach area, do try this routine a few times. The keynote for enjoying it is gradual, deep pressure, with sensitivity. Don't linger on points that feel resistant or uncomfortable; concentrate on the ones where you can penetrate easily and which feel good. Take it slowly and imagine that you are reaching gently deep into your abdomen.

CAUTION

It is not a good idea to do this routine with a full stomach (wait at least an hour after eating) or a full bladder! The routine works best if you are lying on a comfortable but supportive surface (not a sagging bed – a mat or quilt on the floor would be better). You may be more comfortable with your knees raised, but this is not necessary.

CLOCKWISE MASSAGE AROUND LOWER ABDOMEN

Stretch your hands out in front of you, one palm on the back of the other hand, with your fingers overlapped so that you can see all ten fingers side by side. The fingertips of both hands should touch (although if it feels awkward, you can use the fingertips of one hand at a time and alternate as necessary for different abdominal areas). This is your working tool for this sequence.

Place the joined fingertips on the left side of your lower abdomen, in a line along your hip bone. Press around the lower edge of your abdomen in a semicircle up to the top of the right hip. Press straight in as you work around. Cross to the left side again, and press in another semicircle, slightly smaller than the last. If any points feel particularly good, pay special attention to them. Continue pressing in decreasing semicircles until you are just working around your navel. Observe your sensations. Be sensitive.

Lie on a comfortable surface and gradually increase the pressure as you massage around the lower abdomen.

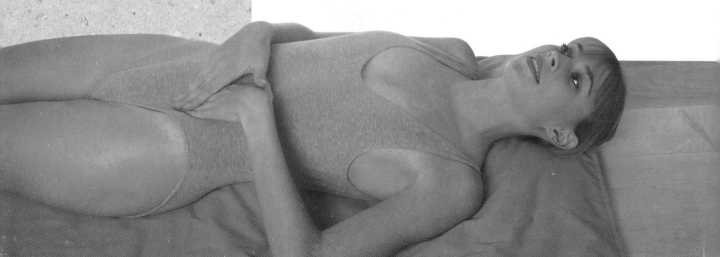

CLOCKWISE MASSAGE AROUND UPPER ABDOMEN

Place the tips of your joined fingers at the top of the left side of your rib cage. Press into the soft tissue along the edge of the rib cage, following it down toward your waist. At waist level, cross over to the right side, and press in a line upward along the edge of the rib cage on the right. Go slowly and gently. If a pressure is uncomfortable, move on – don't continue with it.

When you reach the top, cross over and work down the left side again, a little farther away from the ribs this time. At waist level, cross over to press up the right side, keeping the same distance from the ribs. Keep going in a decreasing pattern until you are working around the top of the navel.

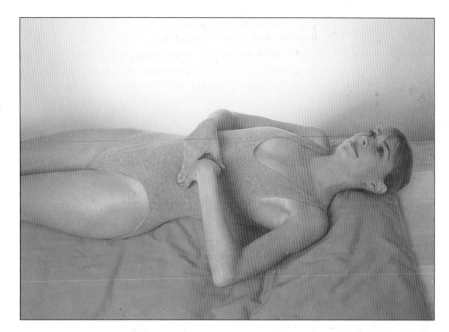

CLOCKWISE CIRCLING

Place one palm over your navel, and put the other hand on top. Relax your hands; let them get heavy and melt into your body. Pressing in very gently, begin to move your joined hands in tiny circles clockwise around your navel. Very gradually increase the size of the circles, keeping your hands on your navel, until you are moving the surface of your abdomen in as big circles as is comfortable. Keep it slow and keep your hands relaxed. Observe your sensations. Traditionally, one does 50 circles, but do as many as you like.

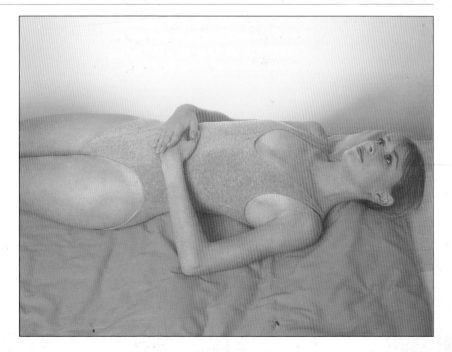

PRESSURES FROM CHEST TO STOMACH

Place your middle finger in the very center of your chest, in the middle of the breastbone. With the fingertips of the other hand, press in a continuous line down from that point (visualizing pressing gently through the bone and without losing awareness of the finger in the middle of your chest), until you find yourself on the softer tissue of the upper abdomen. Keep pressing down in a straight line until you are about halfway between your ribs and your navel.

Don't take your other finger off the center of your chest. Use it as a marker, and now with your other, working hand press with your fingertips in a line down the edge of the breastbone, about half an inch to one side of the first line, and the same length. Then do the same down the other side. *If you are a woman, don't press on the breast tissue.*

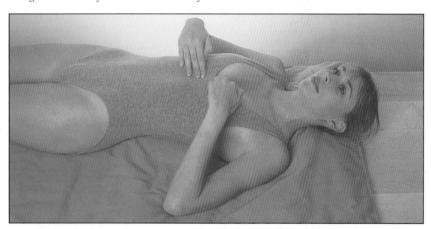

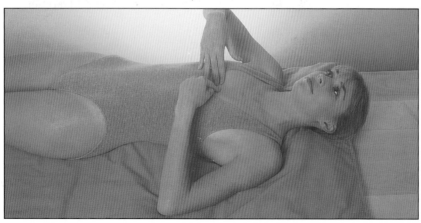

BACK ROUTINE

This routine, suitable for the lower back, is slightly limited by the amount of pressure you can apply with your own thumbs, and by the distance you are able to reach behind you. The routine works best if you are kneeling on a comfortable surface; otherwise, try sitting on a comfortable backless seat such as a piano stool, or astride an ordinary chair, facing its back.

Start with your thumbs as high as you can comfortably reach.

THUMB PRESSURES DOWN SIDES OF SPINE

Reach behind your back until your thumbs are on each side of your spine, as high as you can reach comfortably. Press with your thumbs in lines down both sides of your spine at once, keeping your thumbs level. Press down to hip level. If you find this effective, you can work down your back several times, farther away from the spine each time, so that you cover the whole lower back with vertical lines of pressures.

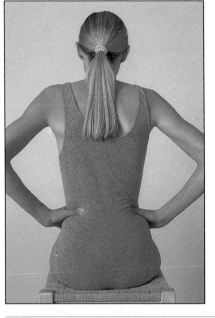

PRESSURES AROUND TOP OF HIP BONES

With your hands on your hips, let your thumbs find the bony ridge of the top of the hip bones and press into the soft tissue just above them, working out from the center and angling your thumbs slightly down to reach under the bone. Work right out to the sides of the hips.

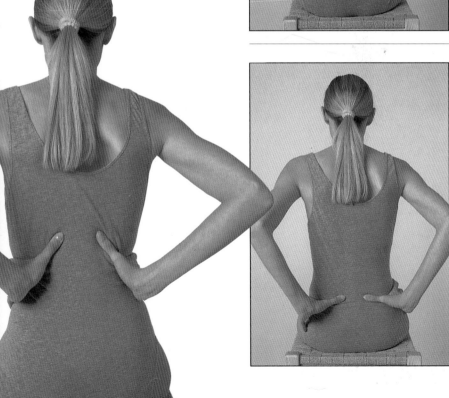

PRESSURES DOWN SACRUM

Still with your hands on your hips, take your thumbs back just to each side of the midline, and move them down onto the flat triangle of bone at the base of your spine (the sacrum). Press with the tips of your thumbs down the sacrum, visualize penetrating deep into your body, and slide your palms farther down the sides of your hips as you press lower. You will find pairs of hollows in a line down the sacrum which are good points to press, but explore and press anywhere that feels good.

ROUTINES WITH A PARTNER

Any of the pressure massage routines described on
pages 26-36 can be adapted to use with a partner, in
combination with the points or by themselves, or in
combination with any other form of massage. Do remember,
when working with a partner, how important it is to relax,
and to use visualization and pressing *beyond* the
surface to increase the effectiveness of your
pressure. Just pressing very hard on the surface
of someone's body *hurts!* It is worthwhile
spending a few seconds to take a couple of
deep breaths before you start; to be aware of
the ground beneath you; to relax your
shoulders and to empty your mind.

*Taking it slowly means that you can
combine a gentle approach with fairly
deep pressure.*

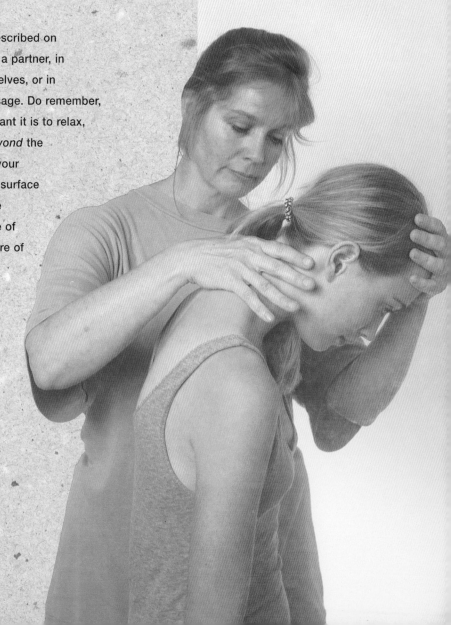

NECK AND SHOULDERS ROUTINE

This routine is one that can be performed anywhere, since your partner sits in a low-backed chair. It is not necessary to remove clothes, although stiff collars, heavy sweaters, or large necklaces and earrings can make things difficult; a soft, loose top or T-shirt is ideal. Make sure your partner's seat is well back on the chair, so that the lower back is supported and he or she does not slump.

GRASPING SHOULDERS AND UPPER ARMS

Place one hand on each of your partner's shoulders. You can do the same grasping movement across her shoulders as you did on yourself (page 32), except that the movement is more effective as you use your thumbs on the back of her shoulders. Stand a short distance from your partner and lean your body weight into your thumbs through straight arms. Continue out to your partner's upper arms.

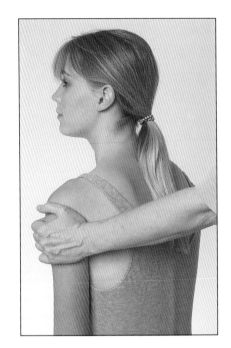

PRESSURES ON UPPER BACK

From the same position as above, move your thumbs to each side of your partner's spine. Lean your body weight in to penetrate beyond the surface of your partner's back. Press in two lines from the top of her back to the level of the bottom of her shoulder blades, then press in two lines outside the first ones until you have covered the area between the shoulder blades. You might like to do some circular movements with your thumbs before you press in if the area is very tense or muscly.

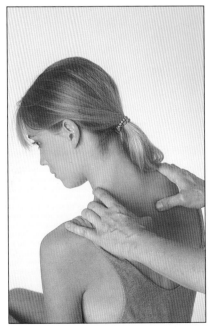

GRASPING UP BACK OF NECK

Stand to the side of your partner and support her forehead with one hand; with the other, hold the back of her neck, thumb on one side, fingers on the other. Squeeze the length of the back of her neck with a grasping movement. This feels so good you will almost certainly be asked to repeat it several times.

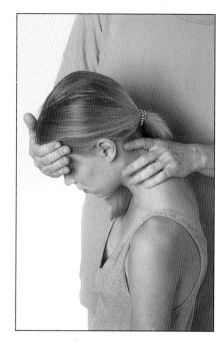

PRESSURES UNDER BASE OF SKULL

In the same position as above, encourage your partner to relax her head forward onto your supporting hand. Find the base of her skull as described on page 30 and press your thumb under it, creating a line of pressure from behind her ear to the back of her neck, and directing your pressure toward the palm of your supporting hand. You will have to change sides to do the other side of her neck with the other thumb.

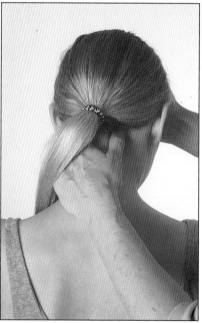

BACK ROUTINE

You have a lot more scope for working on a partner's back than you do on your own, and acupressure can often help chronic back pain. If your partner has back pain of recent onset, however, or if it is very severe, *do make sure a qualified health professional is consulted* to check if it is advisable to give acupressure. For some people, lying on their stomachs can make the back pain worse, and if this is the case, you might start with the Abdominal Routine, which is also helpful for backache, before working on the back. For this routine, it is best if your partner lies on the floor, but put down a mat or quilt or something similar to make it more comfortable.

PRESSURES DOWN THE SIDES OF THE SPINE

Kneel at your partner's side, facing her body. Your partner's arms should be by her sides. (If her neck gets stiff, turning her head from time to time can help). Place one hand gently at the top of her spine, on the side nearest you. Place your other hand an inch or so farther down, still on the side nearest you. Lean your body weight gradually into both your hands, visualizing pressing through your partner to the floor. It is fine if your fingers lie over the spine, as long as you don't press on it. Lean your weight into the heel of the hand and the palm. Keeping the pressure of the upper hand steady, release the lower hand and move it down another 2 inches. Lean your weight into it again. Repeat this procedure all the way down the spine, keeping a continuous, gentle, steady pressure with the top hand and pressing down the side of the spine with your lower hand to just below the waist, where the hip bones start. You may need to move your upper hand down the spine a little as you work farther down. You should be in a crawling position as you lean in. Relax your shoulders!

Then repeat the whole sequence, with the palm of your upper hand resting at the top of the spine as before, and the thumb of the lower hand working into the groove next to the spine on the near side. Support your thumb by placing your fingertips around it so that you can lean your body weight in. When you have pressed the length of your partner's back with your palm and your thumb, cross over to the other side and work down the opposite side of her spine in the same way.

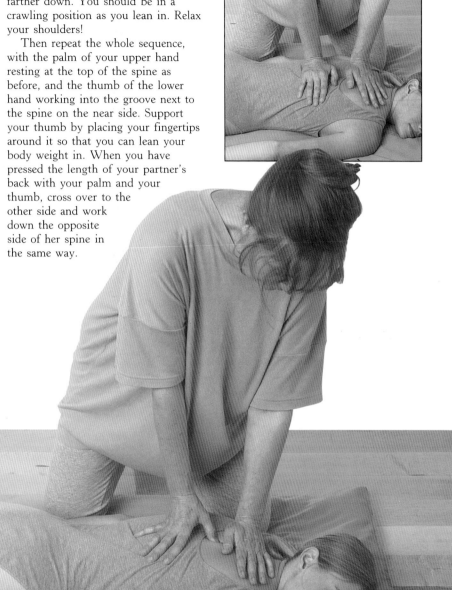

Pressures Down Sacrum

Keep the same position beside your partner as before. Locate the spot where you started to press along her hip bones, but this time move your hands downward. Explore with your fingertips or palms until you find the flat bony triangle at the base of the spine, the sacrum. Supporting your thumbs with your fingertips, lean your body weight into your thumbs to press in two lines down the sacrum, about an inch on each side of the midline. You can lean in with the heels of your hands instead of your thumbs if you prefer. You can also try pressing down the midline and along the edges of the sacrum. This is usually an area where pressure feels good no matter where it is, as long as you lean in gradually with your body weight and penetrate beyond the surface of the body toward the floor.

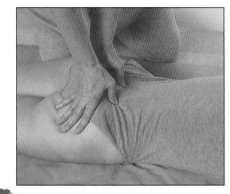

Pressures Around Top of Hip Bones

Kneel beside your partner's hips, facing toward her head. Her arms may be up by her head, or whatever is comfortable, for this and the following movement. Place your hands on each side of her hips, on top of the hip bones, and reach toward the midline with your thumbs so that your thumbs contact the spot where the hip bones start to curve out from the spine, a little below the waist. Press with your thumbs into the soft tissue just above the hip bones, and continue to press in a line outward, following the curve of the bones.

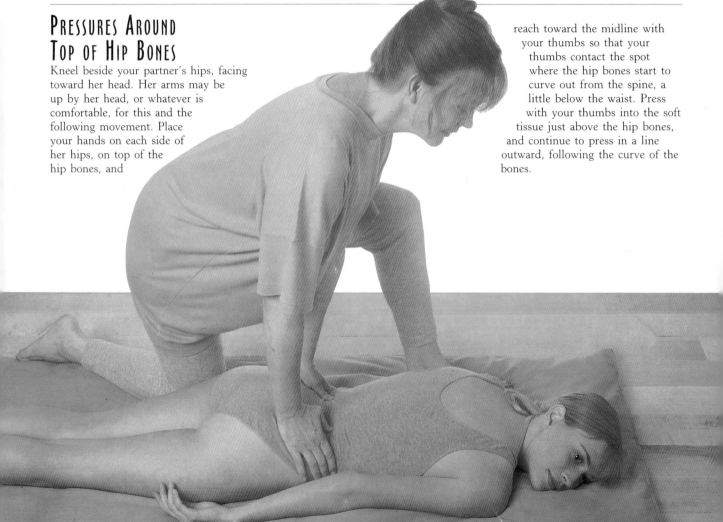

ABDOMINAL ROUTINE

You may need to reassure your partner about how good this can feel (having tried it yourself!) and how effective it is, since many people feel apprehensive about having their stomachs touched. Once again, lying on a mat on the floor is the best position, except that this time your partner is face up. Kneel hip-to-hip with your partner (gently lay his or her nearest arm out to the side so that you can get in close).

PARTNER AWARENESS

Before you start the routine, lay your hand very gently on his or her abdomen and make friendly contact first; be aware of your partner's breathing and make sure you are also aware of your own. Keep your pressure gradual at all times, so that you can release it at once if it is uncomfortable for your partner. If your pressure is gradual, you can go in surprisingly deeply where your partner's comfort allows it. Always be guided by your partner's feedback at all times, and make sure he or she knows that it does not have to hurt to be effective!

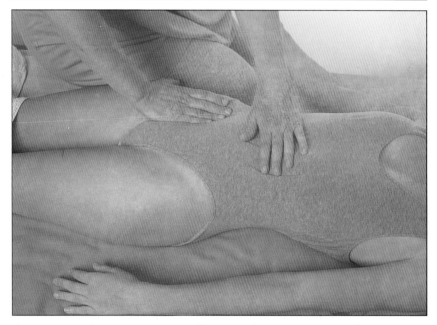

CLOCKWISE PRESSURES AROUND LOWER ABDOMEN

Place one hand gently on your partner's abdomen, above her navel. Place the other hand near her left hip bone and press in slowly and gradually with the flat of your fingertips. Continue with repeated pressures in a semicircle downward next to the bone, then across the lower edge of the abdomen and up next to the right hip bone.

Keep some awareness in the other hand as it rests on the upper abdomen; this is the "listening" hand which will help you tune in to your partner's *Qi*. Do go in deeply where you feel that you can penetrate. At the top of the right hip, cross over again and repeat your pressures in a smaller semicircle, then again in a still smaller one until you reach the area around the navel.

CLOCKWISE PRESSURES AROUND THE UPPER ABDOMEN

Shift your "listening" hand to the area below the navel, and place your other hand on your partner's left side. Either hand can be the "listening" hand, and you can change your hands around whenever you like. With the flat of your fingertips, press gently down beside her rib cage on that side from top to bottom, next to the ribs. At the waistline, cross over to the other side and press up the right-hand side of the rib cage from bottom to top, next to the ribs. Then press down the left side again, but this time an inch or so farther toward the midline. When you cross to the right at the waist, press

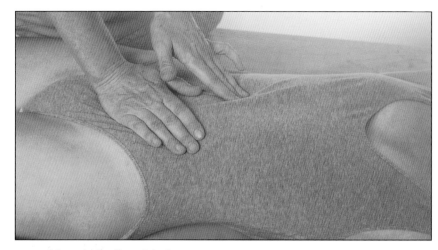

upward in a similar line, 2 inches away from the rib cage. Continue in this way until you have covered the whole upper abdomen and are close to the navel.

ROCKING THE ABDOMEN

Facing your partner's body sideways, place one hand over her navel and the other hand on top of it. With the heels of your hands, gently push your partner's navel area away from you, then with your fingertips draw it back toward you. Repeat this, without moving your hands on the abdominal surface, in a wave-like movement of your hands, so that you are gently rocking the center of your partner's abdomen from side to side. When you stop, rest one hand on the center of the abdomen for a moment, being aware of your partner's breathing.

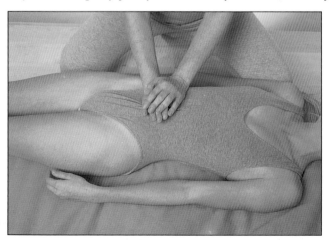

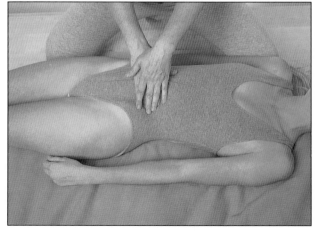

FACE AND HEAD ROUTINE

This is an ultra-relaxing routine; don't be surprised if your partner drifts off to sleep. For this reason, it is nice to combine it with any of the other routines, although in itself it is very effective for tension headaches or sinus congestion. You could do this routine from a kneeling position at the foot of the bed while your partner lies on it, but kneeling behind your partner's head on the floor is better, particularly for the opening movements.

OPENING MOVEMENTS

Place your hands on your partner's shoulders, with your fingers wrapped around the outside of her shoulders and the heels of your hands in the grooves between her shoulders and her chest. Bring your upper body upward and forward, using its weight to flatten your partner's shoulders and open her chest. Hold for a few seconds. Then kneel back again and slide your hands up to the tops of your partner's shoulders. Push your partner's shoulders away from you toward her feet. Slide your hands under your partner's upper back, palms up, and slide them slowly up her back and sides of the neck and off the back of her head. This helps to get long hair away from the neck, but also feels great. Your partner should now already feel relaxed and ready for the face routine.

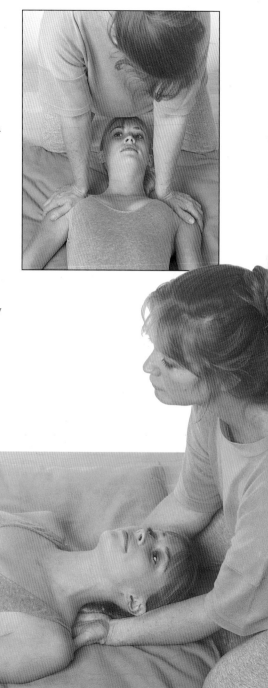

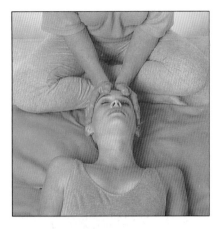

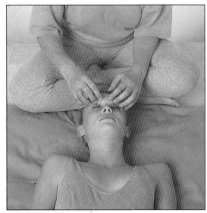

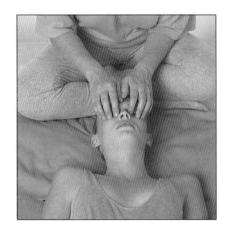

PRESSURES ACROSS THE FOREHEAD

Cup your hands around the sides of your partner's head, and place your thumbs in the space between her eyebrows. With both thumbs pressing gently downward, work out in a line to the temples. Return your thumbs to the midline, slightly higher on her forehead, and repeat. Cover the whole forehead with pressures in this way.

PRESSURES AROUND EYE SOCKETS

Ask your partner to close her eyes. Curl your fingers and place your fingertips lightly around the edge of the bones just below your partner's eyebrows. Use hardly any pressure. Simply feeling for the bone and resting your fingertips along its edge is usually enough. Work from the bridge of the nose out. (You could use your

fingertips separately, as if playing the piano.) The lower edges of the eye sockets lie just below the eyelashes of your partner's closed eyes. Rest your fingertips gently on the edge of the bone.

JAW PRESSURES

Continuing on from the cheek pressures, when you come to the area below the nostrils, press in a semi-circle around the upper jaw to the corners of the mouth. Then rest your fingertips lightly under the chin and use your thumbs to press from the center of the groove under the lower lip out along the jawbone until you

reach the ears, moving the support of your fingertips out and along as you press. When you reach the ears, swap the tips of your middle fingers for your thumbs (it is easier) and press in a line in front of the ears up toward the temples.

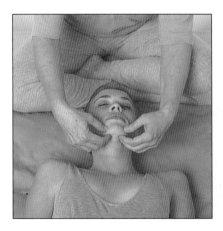

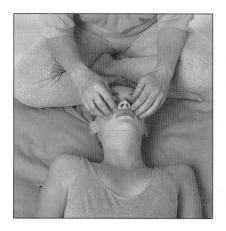

PRESSURES ON CHEEKS

Rest your fingertips on your partner's cheeks, just below the edges of her eye sockets. Working from the sides of the nose toward the ears, press gently in as if toward the back of your partner's head. Cover the whole surface of the cheeks in this way. When you reach the level of the nostrils and the laughter lines, curl your fingertips slightly more and press up under the cheekbones.

SCALP PRESSURES

Cup your hands lightly around the sides of your partner's head and use your thumbs to press in lines along the top of her head, from hairline to crown. Turn your partner's head to one side and support it with one hand. With the thumb of the other hand, cover the side of her head with pressures, starting in a semicircle around the outline of the ear and moving in bigger semicircles outward. Turn her head to the other side and repeat the process. Replace her head in its normal position and finish by running your fingertips through her hair several times from front to back, fingers just touching the scalp.

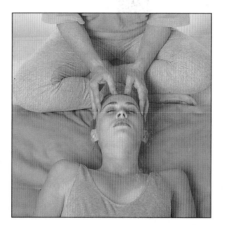

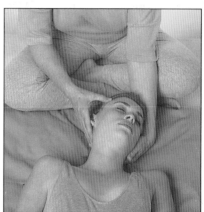

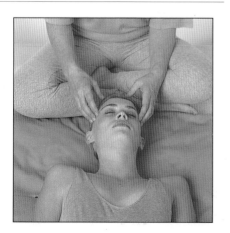

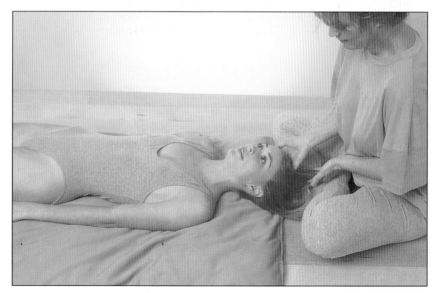

SPECIFIC APPLICATIONS

If you turned to this section first, please read the one on Basic Principles (pages 8-11) before you start looking up treatments for specific conditions. Your acupressure will be far more effective if you work with it according to the principles explained earlier.

As Oriental medicine classifies diseases differently from Western orthodox medicine, ailments can often be due to one of a variety of causes. Wherever space allows, the different forms the ailment can take are given, but occasionally the classifications are too complex for the scope of this book, and a medley of acupressure points is given. All the points are safe to press, however, even if they are not specifically indicated for you. Since Oriental medicine also includes advice on lifestyle, some commonsense health advice is given for some ailments, according to Oriental principles.

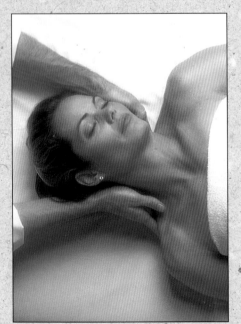

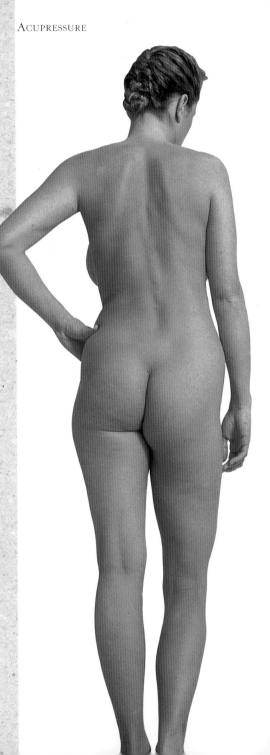

Try to make time to fit in the routines - you'll find them both relaxing and beneficial.

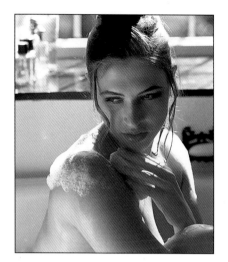

STRESS-RELATED AILMENTS, ACHES, AND PAINS

pages 50–52

Stress is such a widespread condition that it is a factor in many diseases, including many serious pathologies. The more common ones included here are back pain, headache, neck and shoulder tension, chronic fatigue, hangover, anxiety, and insomnia.

DIGESTIVE COMPLAINTS

pages 53–55

Millions of digestive remedies are sold over the counter every year. Acupressure can be very helpful, however, for complaints such as nausea, indigestion, irritable bowel syndrome, constipation, and diarrhea.

RESPIRATORY DISORDERS

pages 56–57

Also on the increase as a result of air pollution are respiratory complaints. This section concentrates on the everyday complaints such as the common cold, cough, hay fever, and sinusitis. The points which help these disorders, however, can also be used safely for more serious respiratory conditions such as asthma. Remember that breathing exercises significantly ease asthma symptoms.

REPRODUCTIVE AND URINARY DISORDERS

pages 58–59

Also commonly known as "women's complaints," these are especially amenable to acupressure treatment. This section examines premenstrual syndrome and menstrual pain, candida (yeast), cystitis, and poor circulation.

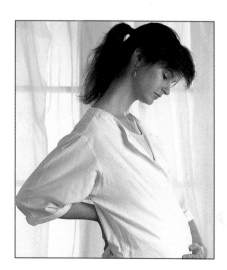

WARNING

Please remember that acupressure is to be used alongside, not instead of, orthodox medical treatment. Your complaint should have been diagnosed by a physician before you decide to use acupressure in addition to any medication prescribed. All points and routines are most effective if done regularly and frequently; at least every other day and preferably every day until symptoms subside. In acute conditions, you can press the points as often as you need to obtain relief, and the routines can be done twice a day.

The Points:
The diagrams show the approximate locations of the points. However, you will need to look up their specific locations on pages 12-25.

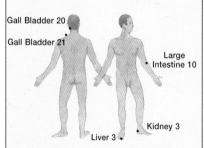

Gall Bladder 20
Gall Bladder 21
Large Intestine 10
Kidney 3
Liver 3

Routines:
It may be harder to find time to do the routines than to press the points, but do try to fit them in.

STRESS-RELATED AILMENTS, ACHES, AND PAINS

Stress is widely recognized in our time as a major cause of disease. The fast pace of living, the constant overload of stimuli to our nervous systems, and the undercurrent of anxiety which runs through the lives of many people all contribute to it. In ancient China, stress was equally present, although often in more dramatic forms such as war and famine. The pace of life was slower, although the level of hardship was greater. Then as now, however, the physician's art was only a supplementary aid. The most effective way to combat stress is to relax our minds and strengthen our core energy; points alone cannot do it.

FATIGUE

Chronic fatigue is on the increase in our society. It can be due to a variety of causes: weak constitution, overwork, poor diet and breathing habits, uneven distribution of *Qi* from emotional stress, or external causes (such as illness) from the past which have been improperly treated and linger in the body. The points below cover all these possibilities.

You should make sure that you are getting the sleep you need, eating moderate and regular cooked meals, and taking some regular, gentle exercise. Tai Chi or Qi Gong are often helpful, as is yoga. In any case, you need to do some deep abdominal breathing every day. Try not to drink lots of coffee or tea to keep you going; it will burn up your resources even more and make you want to drink alcohol to help you relax later, which will stagnate your *Qi* and make you more tired. Royal jelly is a tonic, but don't use ginseng if you have difficulty sleeping: it is "heating." Guarana is another form of caffeine (not many people know this) and should be avoided, like coffee.

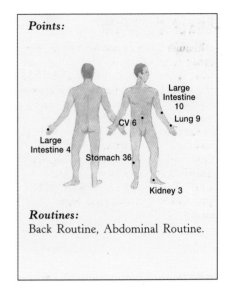

Points:

Large Intestine 10
Lung 9
CV 6
Large Intestine 4
Stomach 36
Kidney 3

Routines:
Back Routine, Abdominal Routine.

HEADACHE

Headaches can be due to a wide variety of causes. If you have a headache because you are tired or tense, the techniques in this book plus some rest and relaxation will help. Sinusitis and hangovers are dealt with on pages 56 and 52. If you have migraines, or very frequent or severe headaches, or have had headaches for a long time, you will need to consult a doctor if you have not already done so, and then see a registered acupressure practitioner. (Acupuncture, herbal remedies, and homeopathy are also helpful for headaches; do find a registered practitioner, though).

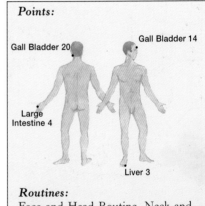

Points:

Gall Bladder 20
Gall Bladder 14
Large Intestine 4
Liver 3

Routines:
Face and Head Routine, Neck and Shoulder Routine, Abdominal Routine.

LOWER BACKACHE

Although lower backache may be the result of an injury, it often gets worse when you are tired and stressed. Take it as a hint from your body that you need to rest. Keep your lower body warm and covered. Abdominal breathing will strengthen your kidneys and back. Avoid strenuous exercise until the pain subsides, but yoga and Tai Chi can be helpful. Be careful when lifting; lift heavy objects with your knees bent and your back straight.

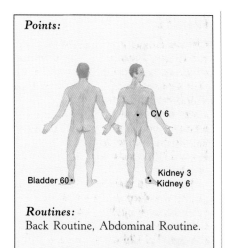

Points:

CV 6

Bladder 60 •

Kidney 3
Kidney 6

Routines:
Back Routine, Abdominal Routine.

NECK AND SHOULDER TENSION

Neck and shoulder tension results from a "top-heavy" distribution of *Qi* and is very common in those who have a sedentary occupation in which they have to concentrate their minds. Try to get *Qi* back to the lower half of your body and legs with some enjoyable exercise such as walking in the park or dancing. Deep, relaxed abdominal breathing can be helpful. If the tension is very bad, you may want to visit an acupressure or Shiatsu practitioner.

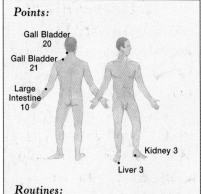

Points:

Gall Bladder 20

Gall Bladder 21

Large Intestine 10

Kidney 3

Liver 3

Routines:
Neck and Shoulder Routine (all the routines can be helpful here, for different reasons; try all of them and see which ones suit you).

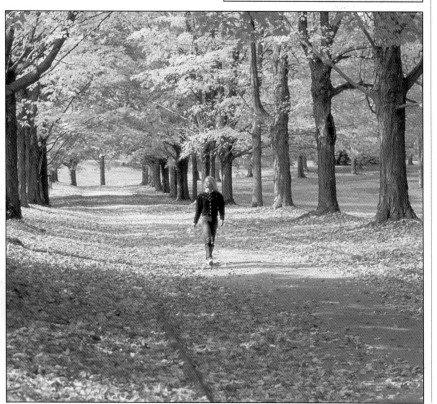

Try to get Qi back to the lower half of your body and legs with some enjoyable exercise such as walking in the park or dancing. Deep, relaxed abdominal breathing can be helpful.

ANXIETY AND INSOMNIA

Chronic anxiety and insomnia are often the result of the kidneys not supplying coolness and relaxation to the *Qi*, so that it gets "hot and bothered." Deep breathing into the lower abdomen is essential for these conditions, as it supports the kidneys.

Sit upright and observe your breathing pattern. It is likely to be fast and shallow. Allow it to be that way for a little while; acknowledge it and keep observing it. It will begin to quieten. Encourage your breath to move downward by expanding your abdomen slightly as you breathe in, contracting it as you breathe out. Visualize the breath flowing down like water to collect in the lower part of your body. Keep observing it, in a friendly and accepting way, not a punishing one; and as you simply watch your breath coming and going, your mind will quieten, too.

This is a simple form of self-help meditation; you can also study other forms, including moving meditations such as yoga and *Tai Chi*. Watching TV is not helpful for insomnia, nor is excessive work on a computer. Eating late at night and drinking large amounts of alcohol are also contra-indicated, although a moderate amount of alcohol may relax you; you will know yourself whether a single drink suits you. If you drink too much, you may need to read the following!

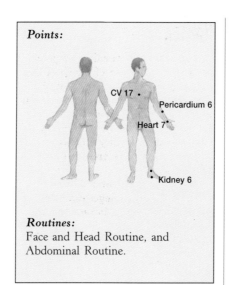

Points:

CV 17

Pericardium 6

Heart 7

Kidney 6

Routines:
Face and Head Routine, and Abdominal Routine.

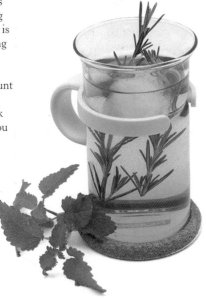

Drink lots of fluids. Herbal teas can help. Try the Japanese drink; green tea – bancha – with a dash of tamari soya sauce.

HANGOVER

There are lots of old wives' tales on how to deal with a hangover, and they are all worth a try. For future reference, vodka and organic wines, or beers are far less likely to give you a hangover! Meanwhile, try a protein-rich breakfast if you can face it, and drink lots of fluids (the Japanese drink green tea – *bancha* – with a dash of tamari soy sauce). If you have any essential oils (see *Aromatherapy* in this series), sniffing undiluted rose or rosemary oil is often helpful. Herbal teas can also help (see *Herbal Remedies* in this series), and Vitamin B (as in yeast tablets) replaces vitamins which the body uses up in dealing with the alcohol.

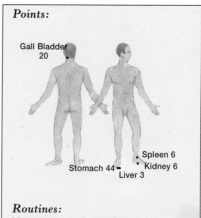

Points:

Gall Bladder 20

Spleen 6

Stomach 44

Kidney 6

Liver 3

Routines:
You may not have the energy to do any of the routines, but if someone can do the Face and Head Routine on you very gently, it will be soothing.

DIGESTIVE COMPLAINTS

Digestive problems are becoming increasingly common, partly because of increasingly stressful lifestyles, partly because of poor eating habits and extreme ideas about diets. Women, particularly, are susceptible because of dieting, often alternated with overeating; according to the Oriental way of thinking, this is a sure way to impair digestion permanently. The foods are also less fresh than they should be, because of processing and preservatives; even "fresh" produce often travels thousands of miles to stores, preserved by irradiation. Stale or processed foods are "wrecked" in terms of *Qi*, and in the long-term overwork the digestive system. Try to eat only fresh, local produce in season if your digestion is weak.

NAUSEA

Nausea results from either temporary or chronic unsettling of the *Qi* of the stomach, or it can be the result of damp, heavy *Qi* from overeating, or an improper diet. If you are able to eat, eat moderate and regular meals. Avoid greasy foods and dairy produce. Chinese or Japanese green tea may also be helpful.

If you are pregnant and have morning sickness, ginger can help, either eaten fresh or in capsule form.

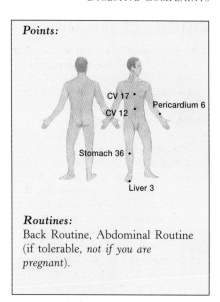

Points:

CV 17
CV 12
Pericardium 6
Stomach 36
Liver 3

Routines:
Back Routine, Abdominal Routine (if tolerable, *not if you are pregnant*).

INDIGESTION

Oriental medicine places great importance on eating habits. Meals should be eaten sitting down, not grabbed on the run. Eating times should be calm and devoted to enjoying the food, not to family bickering, work discussions, reading, or watching TV. (Research has shown that the digestive process does not start until *two hours after* watching TV!) Meals should be regular and moderate; eat some breakfast and don't eat a big meal late at night when your stomach *Qi* is low. Very importantly, foods should be cooked, not raw. Avoid fatty, greasy foods.

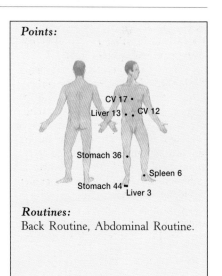

Points:

CV 17
Liver 13
CV 12
Stomach 36
Spleen 6
Stomach 44
Liver 3

Routines:
Back Routine, Abdominal Routine.

IRRITABLE BOWEL SYNDROME

According to Oriental medical principles, this condition is the result of emotional stress combined with a weak digestion. It is very common these days. Eat warm, cooked foods; avoid cold drinks and spicy food. Drink alcohol and coffee in moderation or not at all. Deep abdominal breathing, moderate and enjoyable exercise, and above all relaxation are all helpful.

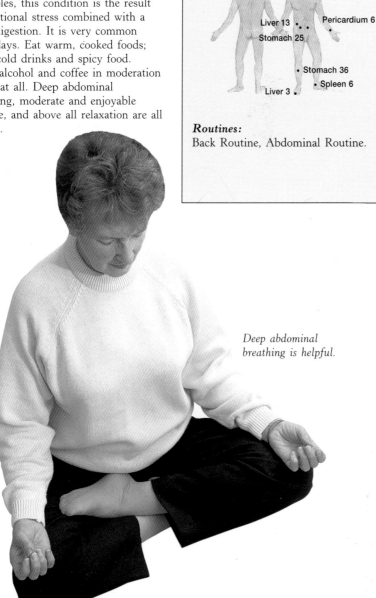

Deep abdominal breathing is helpful.

Points:

Liver 13
Pericardium 6
Stomach 25
Stomach 36
Spleen 6
Liver 3

Routines:
Back Routine, Abdominal Routine.

CONSTIPATION

According to Oriental medicine, constipation can often be the result of emotional "holding" transferred to the digestive process. Relaxation is important, combined with deep breathing to massage the abdominal organs from inside and moderate, enjoyable exercise.

Contrary to modern Western fashion, don't go overboard on raw fruits and vegetables; cooked grains and lightly cooked vegetables provide just as much fiber and do not strain your digestive system, which has to turn everything you eat into gastric soup. Make sure you drink enough liquid, but don't overdo it! Four or five cups a day (not all coffee!) is ample: more only if you are thirsty. Avoid spices, which may help in the short term but ultimately make the problem worse.

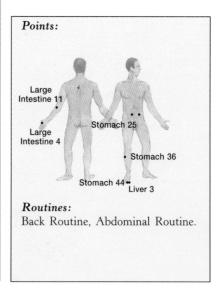

Points:

Large Intestine 11
Large Intestine 4
Stomach 25
Stomach 36
Stomach 44
Liver 3

Routines:
Back Routine, Abdominal Routine.

DIARRHEA

If your diarrhea is acute and the result of a temporary stomach upset, rest and drink plenty of fluids. In India, white rice, natural live yogurt, and black tea are recommended for acute diarrhea.

Consult your doctor if it has not cleared up after 48 hours, or is very severe. Consult your doctor immediately if a child has diarrhea.

If the diarrhea is chronic (i.e., permanently loose stools), Oriental medicine diagnoses dampness and a weak digestion. Help your digestion to function normally by feeding it cooked, warm foods. Avoid very cold drinks. Eat breakfast! Keep warm! Take regular, moderate exercise.

The best form of exercise to go with acupressure is Tai Chi or Qi Gong, which work directly on the Qi.

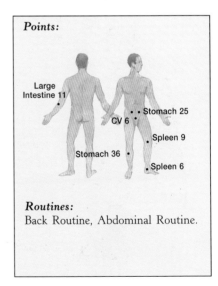

Points:

Large Intestine 11

CV 6

Stomach 25

Spleen 9

Stomach 36

Spleen 6

Routines:
Back Routine, Abdominal Routine.

RESPIRATORY DISORDERS

In the Oriental medical system, colds and flu are considered to be the result of wind or damp penetrating the body and affecting the lungs. Depending on a person's constitution, some people are more prone to wind, some to damp, but it is best to avoid both.

COUGH

If you have a phlegmy cough, you should avoid consuming dairy products. For all coughs, get as much rest as you can and do the breathing exercise on page 52. Cover yourself up well when it is cold, and avoid the sun in summer. Inhale steam from a bowl of boiling water to loosen mucus and soothe the lungs. You can add appropriate essential oils (see *Aromatherapy* in this series).

Points:

Lung 1   CV 22
CV 17
Lung 5
Lung 7
Lung 9
Stomach 36
Spleen 6
Kidney 6

Routines:
Neck and Shoulder Routine, Back Routine.

SINUSITIS

Mucus and phlegm are often linked to improper diet. Avoid dairy products, peanuts, and bananas, which all encourage the secretion of mucus, and severely limit alcohol, coffee, and hot or spicy foods, which make the mucus thick and sticky.

Inhale steam from a bowl of boiling water; add some menthol or essential oil to the water for extra effect.

Points:

Bladder 2
Large
Intestine 20
Stomach 3
Large
Intestine 4
Stomach 36
Spleen 6

Routines:
Face and Head Routine, Abdominal Routine.

COMMON COLD

At the very beginning of a cold, the repeated use of these points may avert the cold completely, if you combine them with a soothing hot drink or any other folk remedy you may know that causes sweating, and go to bed and keep warm.

If the cold still takes hold, keep warm and *rest!* A cold is an illness, even though a common one, and your body needs energy to fight it off. Only take antibiotics or cold-suppressants as a last resort. Do the Neck and Shoulder Routine and the Face and Head Routine for symptomatic relief, and continue to press the points below for speedy recovery.

Points:

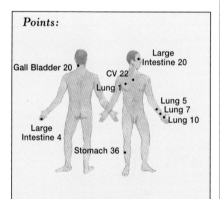

Gall Bladder 20
Large Intestine 20
CV 22
Lung 1
Lung 5
Lung 7
Lung 10
Large Intestine 4
Stomach 36

If you have a sore throat, use Lung 10 and CV 22. If you have a phlegmy cough or wheeze, use Lung 1 and 5. If your nose is runny or blocked, use Large Intestine 4 and 20.

HAY FEVER

Hay fever, which used to be a seasonal problem related to pollen, is now a permanent condition for many people. If it is seasonal, use the symptomatic points and routines when the problem is active, and the long-term points and routines for the rest of the year. If it is a permanent condition, use all the points plus Neck and Shoulder Routine and Abdominal Routine.

Points for relief of symptoms:

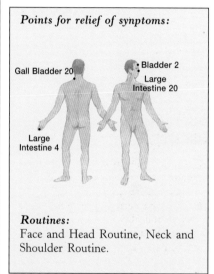

Gall Bladder 20
Bladder 2
Large Intestine 20
Large Intestine 4

Routines:
Face and Head Routine, Neck and Shoulder Routine.

Hay fever, although triggered by inhaling certain irritants, is often linked to long-standing chronic allergies to some food substance. If there is any food or drink which you crave in large quantities, beware! You are likely to be allergic to it. See if your symptoms improve if you cut it out of your diet for a week (go on, try!).

Points for long-term treatment of underlying condition:

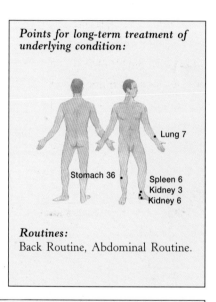

Lung 7
Stomach 36
Spleen 6
Kidney 3
Kidney 6

Routines:
Back Routine, Abdominal Routine.

PREVENTATIVE MEASURES

Wrap your neck and head if it is windy, or when riding a bicycle or motorbike. Avoid drafts and air-conditioning where possible. Don't wander about with wet hair after swimming or showering; dry it as soon as possible. And wrap yourself up after exercise or a hot bath, as you are more vulnerable when your pores are open.

Most people who live in cities are susceptible to the effects of air pollution and need to pay special attention to strengthening their lungs with breathing exercises. A simple exercise is given under Anxiety on page 52, but you can learn other techniques at yoga or *Qi Gong* classes. Research has shown that the majority of asthma sufferers can control or alleviate their symptoms with breathing exercises.

REPRODUCTIVE AND URINARY DISORDERS

Acupressure is extremely effective for women's complaints, many of which are labeled as "psychosomatic" by Western medicine if there is no obvious pathology present. Oriental medicine, on the other hand, respects the link between the emotions and the body, and treats it through the *Qi*, the interface where the physical and the emotional meet. In women, this link manifests in the delicate hormonal balance of the menstrual cycle, and acupressure is a safe and effective way of restoring or maintaining that balance.

PRE-MENSTRUAL SYNDROME (PMS)

Press the points every day, not just when you are pre-menstrual. Coffee is known to contribute to PMS and menstrual pain (in Oriental medical terms, it causes stagnation of *Qi*), so try to cut down on it. Vitamin supplements and evening primrose oil are helpful for many women.
If you are prone to PMS, make a note in your diary of the time when you are likely to start experiencing it, and try to avoid overloading your schedule. Allow time for yourself and your feelings. The menstrual period throughout the Far East is considered a time for a woman to be quiet and reflect, a time when she is especially sensitive and perceptive, so allow it to be a "different" time for you, and take it a bit easy.

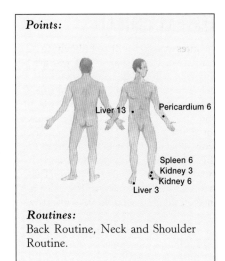

Points:

Liver 13 . | Pericardium 6

Spleen 6
Kidney 3
Kidney 6
Liver 3

Routines:
Back Routine, Neck and Shoulder Routine.

MENSTRUAL PAIN

Throughout the East, cold is considered to contribute substantially to menstrual pain. If you have menstrual pain, especially pain that is eased by a hot-water bottle, it is best to avoid ice cream and cold foods for the week before your period, and avoid getting your lower body cold (i.e., sitting in a damp swimsuit, or with a draft on your lower back, or sitting on a cold surface).

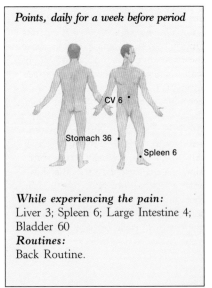

Points, daily for a week before period

CV 6 .

Stomach 36 .

. Spleen 6

While experiencing the pain:
Liver 3; Spleen 6; Large Intestine 4; Bladder 60
Routines:
Back Routine.

YEAST (CANDIDA)

Acupressure by itself is unlikely to cure a yeast infection, but if you are prone to it, regular acupressure will help prevent attacks. You should be careful not to eat raw or cold foods, and cut down on dairy products except for live yogurt. Ginger (fresh, stir-fried with vegetables) is a good addition to the diet. Wear cotton panties, and stockings rather than pantyhose. Tea-tree oil is available as suppositories and in creams which can be very effective.

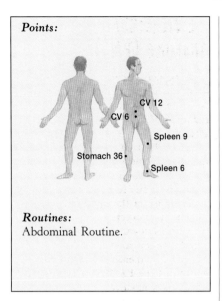

Points:

CV 12
CV 6
Spleen 9
Stomach 36
Spleen 6

Routines:
Abdominal Routine.

POOR CIRCULATION

Deep breathing and moderate regular exercise will both help greatly. *Qi Gong* in particular is a wonderful circulation booster, if done regularly. Cut down on coffee and cigarettes, and eat lots of ginger. Several essential oils improve the circulation when added to the bath water or massaged into the skin (see *Aromatherapy* in this series). Skin brushing (from the extremities toward the heart) improves the circulation; a stronger method, if you don't have sensitive skin, is to put a thick layer of salt on a damp washcloth (the mitt kind is easiest) and to rub the skin with it after a bath or shower, adding more salt as necessary. Avoid cuts, and sensitive areas such as the face and genitals, and rinse off well with tepid water.

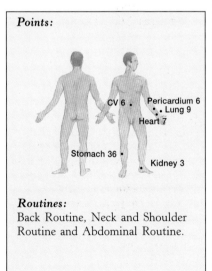

Points:

CV 6
Pericardium 6
Lung 9
Heart 7
Stomach 36
Kidney 3

Routines:
Back Routine, Neck and Shoulder Routine and Abdominal Routine.

CYSTITIS

You should press these points daily, not just when you have cystitis. *You should always see a doctor if you have a fever, back pain, or blood in your urine.* However, cystitis can often be cured by keeping warm, resting, and drinking lots of fluids to flush out the infection. Herbs can be very effective – check *Herbal Remedies* in this series for some herbs that may help. You should always wear cotton underwear, stockings rather than pantyhose, and wipe from front to back after urinating. White wine and non-organic beer often contain chemicals that irritate a sensitive bladder, so avoid them if possible. It is not uncommon for cystitis to be related to sexual intercourse, if there is an element of fear or insecurity in the relationship; this may be something to consider.

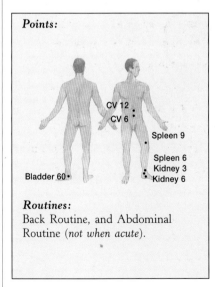

Points:

CV 12
CV 6
Spleen 9
Spleen 6
Kidney 3
Kidney 6
Bladder 60

Routines:
Back Routine, and Abdominal Routine (*not when acute*).

Consulting a Practitioner

Acupressure is capable of treating many more conditions than can be described in a book of this length. If, for example, you have arthritis or rheumatism, or want to help a friend who has it, there are techniques and points suitable for treating every joint in the body, and there is not enough space here to list them all. If you are interested in studying further, you will need to contact the relevant professional society (addresses opposite) for a list of approved schools or training programs. Most schools offer introductory courses which will help you to treat family and friends without undertaking a full professional training program.

Many styles of acupressure are now practiced in the West, some very vigorous, others more similar to spiritual healing, some working with meridians, others with points, some working through clothes, others on bare skin, some completely off the body. Many have incorporated other forms of healing, and most have abandoned the Western name of "acupressure," so that looking for a practitioner can become confusing. Some of the styles are described below:

Shen Tao Acupressure on points alone, only a few points at a session, on bare skin. Very gentle.

Tui-Na Traditional Chinese massage incorporating acupuncture points, usually on bare skin. Vigorous and dynamic.

Namikoshi (or *Nippon Shiatsu*) Whole body routine, usually through clothes, with specific combinations of points for specific ailments. This is the version of Shiatsu most often found in Japan. Incorporates some stretches. Vigorous.

Zen Shiatsu The whole body is treated through clothes, following meridians and concentrating on points relevant to the receiver's condition. Strong intuitive component with the emphasis on contact with receiver's *Qi*. Incorporates some stretches. Can be vigorous or gentle.

Healing-Shiatsu (Similar to *Zen Shiatsu*) Meditational emphasis in training. Tends to be gentle.

Shiatsu-Do Whole-body routine through clothes, using meridians and

An acupressure or Shiatsu treatment is a relaxing yet invigorating experience.

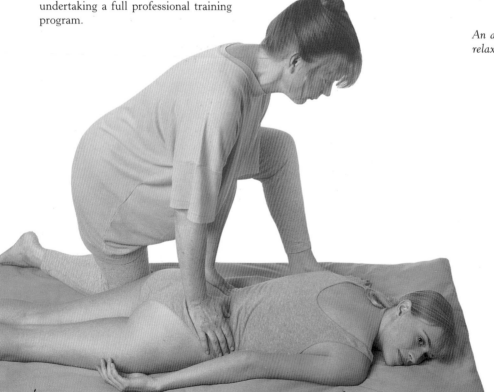

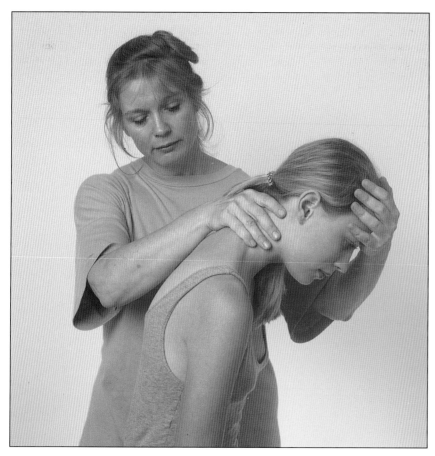

points. More stretches and movement than in *Zen Shiatsu*. Tends to be vigorous and dynamic.

Movement Shiatsu Aims to help chronic postural and emotional problems. In style it is more like the Alexander technique or Feldenkrais method than traditional acupressure, although it works with the meridian system. It uses light pressure on points, gentle manipulations, and guided movement to bring awareness to energy patterns in the body and to resolve inner conflicts.

You may wish to experience what

All registered practitioners of acupressure have completed a thorough training, usually of several years' duration.

acupressure feels like for yourself, in which case you will need to find a practitioner. When looking for a practitioner of acupressure or Shiatsu, first contact the relevant professional society where possible, since it will refer you to a practitioner who has been recognized as competent to a standard accepted by an external board of examiners.

Useful Addresses

Professional body:
American Oriental Bodywork
 Therapy Association
50 Maple Place
Manhasset
New York 11030

American Massage Therapy
 Association
820 Davis Street, Suite 100
Evanston, IL 60201
Tel: 708-8640123

Training:
Pauline Sasaki
151A Scribner Ave
Norwalk
Connecticut 06854

Kiku Miyazaki
Boston Shiatsu School
1815 Massachusetts Ave
Cambridge
Massachusetts

Reading List

Ted Kaptchuk, *Chinese Medicine; The Web That Has No Weaver* (Century, 1985).

Master Lam Kam Chuen, *The Way of Energy* (Gaia Books, 1991).

Lucinda Lidell and others, *The Book of Massage* (Ebury Press, 1984).

Paul Lundberg, *The Book of Shiatsu* (Gaia Books, 1992).

Ed. Dr. Andrew Stanway, *The Natural Family Doctor* (Promotional Reprint Co., 1993).

INDEX

Note: Page numbers in *italics* refer to illustrations.

AKNOWLEDGMENTS

Japan Archive 5, Kevin Phillips/Ace 6,
Image Select 7.
All other photographs are the copyright
of Quarto Publishing plc.

Quarto would like to thank Sarah
Dorin from MOT Model Agency.

Quarto would also like to thank Paul
Crompton for the picture on page 55.